ABOUT THIS BOOK

This book contains four tailored workouts program for anybody who wants to start their pilate journey. Each program is easy to follow since it has **COLORED PICTURES FOR EACH EXERCISE**, clear explanations of **How to Perform Poses**, **suggestions To Avoid Common Mistakes** and General Tips about each exercise.

You will find useful info about Pilates and its benefits, some nutrition advice. All the chapters in this book have been written to help you achieve optimum health and wellbeing.

You can practice one program at the time and when you feel comfortable with the exercises, move to the next one. The key to success with these Wall Pilates Program is to be patient, practice at your own pace and stay consistent, till you are ready to complete a 28-days program.

Please note: if you are a senior beginner there are other books produced by me suitable for you.

What is 28-days program? It will be explained in the next chapters.

If you have any question, you can contact me at:
ritadavis.pilates@gmail.com

DISCLAIMER

This information is for your personal use ONLY. You cannot distribute, copy, reproduce, or otherwise sell this product or information in any form whatsoever, including but not limited to: electronic, or mechanical, including photocopying, recording, or by any informational storage or retrieval system without expressed written, dated and signed permission from the author. All copyrights are reserved.

The information, including but not limited to, text, graphics, images and other material contained in this guide are for informational purposes only. No material from this guide is intended to be a substitute for professional medical advice, diagnosis or treatment.

Always seek the advice of your physician or other qualified health care provider with any questions you may have regarding a medical condition or treatment and before undertaking a new health care regimen, and never disregard professional medical advice or delay in seeking it because of something you have read in this guide.

**"Take care of your body.
It's the only place where you have to live!"**

Jim Rohn

TABLE OF CONTENTS

INTRODUCTION

Wall Pilates is a unique form of exercise that originated in Germany during the late 19th century. It was developed by Joseph H. Pilates, who believed that the physical, mental and spiritual elements of the body should all be connected and in harmony with one another.

Joseph Pilates was a pioneer of his time and wanted to create an exercise that focused on improving strength, posture and flexibility. He developed Wall Pilates as a combination of western and eastern exercise disciplines that focused on targeting the body's deep muscles, connecting them to each other and strengthening them as one unit.

Unlike the typical mat-based Pilates class, wall Pilates uses wall bars to give an even more precise approach to strengthening and sculpting the body. It focuses on pushing and pulling exercises and movement drills which helps create balance, power, agility and stamina. This approach helps to engage the body's core muscles, enhance muscular coordination and create fluid, controlled movements.

By targeting the body's smaller muscles with wall Pilates, it also helps improve posture, boost energy levels and helps reduce aches and pains. It also creates long lasting body changes and improved quality of movement that you can carry with you through everyday activities and workouts.

Joseph Pilates developed wall Pilates more than 100 years ago, but the unique approach and benefits it offers to those who practice it have made it increasingly popular around the world.

The goal of this book is not just to help you learn and understand more about wall Pilates, but to also help you become healthier by getting you to move through the exercise routines that we'll present to you. Your wellbeing is very important to us, and we want to make sure that you have everything you need to maintain your best physical and mental shape. With the information we share with you in this book, you're going to fall back in love with your body, mind and health. You're going to live a healthier and more fulfilling life. And this is what it's all about. We only live once, and we have to make it count.

My youngest daughter Rose helped me throughout the creation fo this book and since she is a beginner with most of these exercises, she is the perfect example for everybody to get started with this simple Wall Pilates Routines.

AUTHORS BIO

Rita Davis is a personal trainer with over 20 years of experience who specializes in senior workouts and has a passion for Nutrition, Yoga, Pilates, and Mindfulness. Rita has dedicated her career to helping people at any age stay healthy and active through safe and effective exercise programs and personalized nutrition plans.

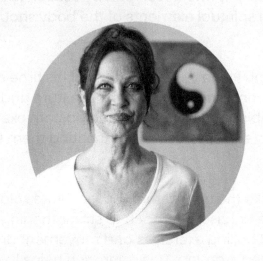

In addition to her work as a personal trainer, Rita is an experienced Pilates and Yoga instructor who incorporates exercises into her clients' workouts to improve their strength, flexibility, and posture.

Rita's passion for health and wellness extends beyond fitness. She provides her clients with valuable nutrition advice and guidance to support their fitness goals. In her free time, practices mindfulness, which she believes is essential for managing stress and promoting overall well-being.

TAKE CARE OF
YOUR BODY AND MIND

As a personal trainer specializing in Pilates workouts for beginners, seniors, and women, I have a deep passion for helping people of all ages and backgrounds achieve their fitness goals. However, it's important to remember that taking care of our bodies and minds is not just about physical exercise - it's a holistic practice.

In our life, it's essential to prioritize our health and wellbeing by paying attention to both our physical and mental health. Pilates is an excellent form of exercise for people of all fitness levels, as it helps develop core strength, improves flexibility and posture, and increases overall body awareness.

Moreover, Pilates can also promote mindfulness and emotional wellbeing by helping us become more present in the moment and reducing stress.

In addition to Pilates, there are other ways to take care of our minds and bodies, such as mindfulness practices, meditation, or yoga.

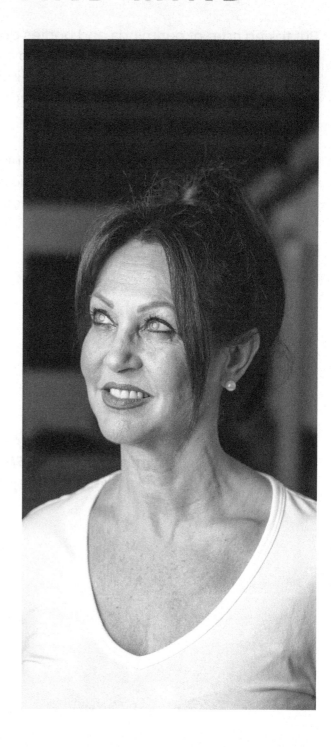

These practices have proven benefits for mental health, including reducing stress and anxiety, improving sleep quality, and promoting relaxation and calmness.

But taking care of our minds and bodies doesn't just involve physical exercise or mindfulness. Social connections are also essential for our overall wellbeing. Participating in group fitness classes or finding a workout buddy can help us stay motivated and connected with others, leading to new friendships and a sense of community.

In conclusion, as a personal trainer, my mission is to help my clients achieve their fitness goals while also promoting holistic health and wellbeing. By prioritizing Pilates, mindfulness practices, and social connections, we can maintain our physical and mental health as we age."

"Exercise not only keeps us fit, but gives us strength, stamina and spirit. Stay active, stay healthy and make your senior years your golden years!"

WHAT IS WALL PILATES?

Wall Pilates is a wonderful way to enhance your physical routine. Designed to strengthen, stretch, and balance the body, this low-impact form of exercise is ideal for those seeking an extra dimension of activity. The exercises in Wall Pilates are done using the wall for resistance, and can include a variety of poses that challenge the entire body. From simple stretches to intense exercises like push-ups, hip thrusts, sit-ups, planks, stretches, balance poses, and more, Wall Pilates is a fantastic way to improve your overall fitness.

Wall Pilates is a great choice for all ages and can be adapted to suit each person's ability level. it is gentle form of exercising and can be customized to suit any age or ability. In addition to improving posture, flexibility, and strength, Wall Pilates can also help reduce stress and fatigue. One of the many advantages of this exercise is that seniors may find it easier to continue with Wall Pilates, as it requires minimal equipment and can be done from the comfort of their own home.

At any age, it's crucial to prioritize our health and wellbeing. As we age, we become more aware of the effects of our past choices on our current state of health. While some choices may have been beneficial, others may have been detrimental. However, it's never too late to make positive changes. This book is meant to guide you through safe and effective workout routines that will help you feel stronger, happier, and more independent. We're here to help you every step of the way.

In the following pages, we will explore wall Pilates in more detail and show you how to get the most out of your workout. So, if you're looking for a safe and effective way to enhance your physical activity, consider trying Wall Pilates.

IS WALL PILATES WORKOUT EFFECTIVE?

Wall Pilates is a unique form of exercise that involves using an exercise wall or sling wall as a key part of the workout. Unlike traditional Pilates, which is typically floor-based, Wall Pilates focuses on using wall-assisted movement to improve flexibility, coordination, strength, and balance. This makes it an accessible and gentle introduction to Pilates for those new to the discipline.

The origins of Wall Pilates can be traced back to Germany in the late 1920s, when Joseph Pilates used pulley systems suspended from walls and ceilings to create his famous exercises. Since then, wall-assisted exercise has been extensively studied and is believed to offer therapeutic benefits in various contexts, including the elderly and post-rehabilitative care.

One of the main benefits of wall Pilates is that it can improve strength, flexibility, and mobility, while also providing relief from back pain. Studies have shown that wall Pilates can be effective for people of all ages, fitness levels, and abilities, including those undergoing physical rehabilitation.

In addition to these physical benefits, wall Pilates can also improve coordination and balance by challenging the body with dynamic movements and changing positions while using the wall for support. By engaging multiple body parts simultaneously, wall Pilates can also help with joint flexibility, strength, and endurance, while reducing tension in the shoulders and hips.

Overall, Wall Pilates has the potential to be widely adopted as an alternative form of exercise due to its popularity and the numerous benefits it offers for people of all fitness levels. While further research is needed to fully understand the specific effects and applications of wall Pilates, it is clear that this form of exercise can help people achieve better health and wellness.

WHY IS WALL PILATES GOOD FOR EVERYBODY ?

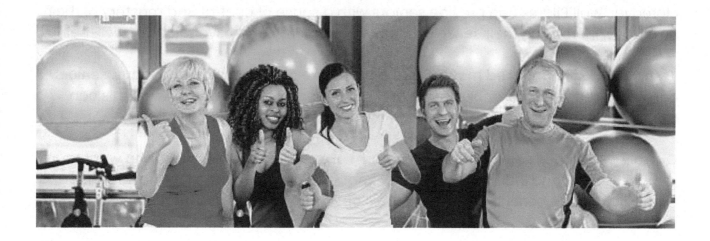

Wall Pilates is a versatile and accessible form of exercise that can benefit people of all ages, fitness levels, and abilities. However, it can be especially valuable for older adults who may be experiencing age-related physical challenges. By focusing on balance, core strength, and proper body alignment, wall Pilates can help seniors maintain their physical fitness and independence.

One of the key benefits of wall Pilates for seniors is that it is low-impact and can be adapted to each individual's ability. This means that seniors can safely engage in wall Pilates even if they have arthritis, mobility impairments, or other age-related issues.

The routine of wall Pilates is often different each day and can include challenging, yet rewarding, exercises that work multiple parts of the body. By using all the muscles in the body instead of isolated movements, seniors can benefit from increased muscular endurance, stability, and flexibility.

Another advantage of wall Pilates for seniors is that it can help increase energy and overall strength. By focusing on core strength, wall Pilates can make everyday activities like walking, climbing stairs, and getting in and out of a chair more efficient and easier.

It can also improve flexibility and range of motion, so older adults can enjoy an increased ability to perform their everyday activities. In addition, wall Pilates can have a calming effect by increasing the awareness of breathing and reducing stress levels, promoting relaxation and reducing anxiety.

Moreover, wall Pilates can provide seniors with a sense of control and mastery of their own body, increasing their sense of physical autonomy and psychological well-being.

By engaging in controlled movements that require concentration and focus, seniors can feel a sense of accomplishment and confidence in their own abilities. This can translate to increased self-esteem and a more positive outlook on life.

Overall, wall Pilates can be an excellent form of exercise for everybody who want to remain healthy and independent. Its low impact exercises, controlled movements, and numerous health benefits make it an ideal option for seniors of all fitness levels and abilities.

BENEFITS OF WALL PILATES

Wall Pilates has taken the world by storm, gaining popularity over the past decade as a unique exercise system that utilizes the support of a wall to improve overall strength and mobility. This innovative form of Pilates provides a wide array of physical and mental benefits, offering something for everyone. Whether you're looking to improve balance, core strength, or simply reduce stress levels, wall Pilates has something to offer. In this chapter, we'll delve deeper into the 10 surprising health benefits of wall Pilates, and explore how it can enhance your life both physically and mentally.

STRENGTHENS THE FULL BODY

Wall Pilates is a powerful and dynamic exercise system that offers a unique and engaging full-body workout. By utilizing the support of a wall, you can engage and strengthen all major muscle groups, from your shoulders and arms to your core, legs, and feet. Unlike traditional workouts, wall Pilates offers a stable surface for you to press into, which allows for greater muscle engagement and faster results.

What's more, wall Pilates offers a variety of exercises that can be easily modified to suit your individual fitness level. Whether you're a beginner or a more advanced exerciser, wall Pilates can help you reach your goals.

These low-impact exercises not only help strengthen and tone your muscles, but also reduce the risk of joint strain or injury.

Additionally, wall Pilates offers a unique and rewarding workout experience that can help boost your mental and emotional well-being. By focusing on controlled movements and breath work, wall Pilates can help reduce stress levels and promote relaxation.

Overall, wall Pilates is an excellent exercise system for anyone looking to improve their strength.

IMPROVES POSTURE

Wall Pilates isn't just another exercise routine. It's a transformative experience that can help improve your overall well-being. One of the most significant benefits of this unique form of Pilates is its ability to promote good posture.

By regularly engaging in wall Pilates exercises, you can strengthen and tone your core, back, and abdomen muscles, which are essential for good posture. It also promotes spinal flexibility, which further contributes to better posture. These exercises are designed to strengthen weak muscles and stretch tight ones, improving your posture over time.

Moreover, wall Pilates is great for spinal alignment, especially when it comes to leg exercises.

Pushing your lower back into the wall while engaging your abs to maintain a neutral spine position helps to keep your spine straight and your posture perfect. Overall, incorporating wall Pilates into your fitness routine can lead to significant improvements in your posture, making you stand taller and feel more confident. Not to mention, it also helps to keep your muscles strong and healthy. So why not give it a try and see how it transforms your posture and overall well-being?

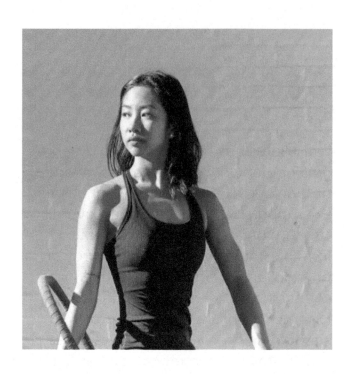

STRENGTHENS THE CORE

Wall Pilates is an effective way to strengthen your core muscles, including the abdominals, back muscles, and hip muscles. By regularly practicing wall Pilates, you can build a stronger core, improve overall body stability and strength, and reduce the risk of injury during everyday activities. Wall Pilates also provides an excellent opportunity to stretch and tone your abdominal muscles, which can help support your lower back and improve your posture. Plus, the wall provides resistance to your movements, which further challenges your core muscles and makes your workout more effective. Incorporating wall Pilates into your fitness routine can help you achieve a stronger, healthier body.

TONES THE ARMS AND LEGS

Wall Pilates is a fantastic way to tone your body and strengthen your major muscle groups. With the use of the wall for support, you can perform various exercises that target your arms and legs, helping you to achieve a lean and toned physique. For example, the pike press exercise engages your arms, chest, and legs, while wall squats help to target your legs and glutes. These moves are designed to challenge your muscles and improve your overall strength and endurance. Best of all, Wall Pilates is a low-impact form of exercise, making it an excellent choice for anyone looking for a safe and effective workout. With regular practice, you'll soon see your muscles becoming more toned and defined, giving you the confidence to take on any challenge that comes your way.

LOW-IMPACT WORKOUT

Looking for a low-impact, yet effective workout? Look no further than Wall Pilates! This form of exercise requires minimal equipment and can easily be done in the comfort of your own home. Unlike many high-impact workouts that can cause stress on your joints, Wall Pilates is gentle on your body, making it ideal for those who suffer from joint pain or injury. It's also perfect for beginners who are just starting their fitness journey, as it allows them to build strength and tone up without overexerting themselves. With Wall Pilates, you can enjoy a full-body workout that will leave you feeling strong and energized, without the risk of injury. Give it a try and see how it can transform your body and your overall well-being!

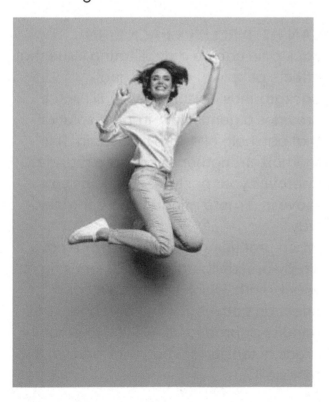

CAN HELP WITH WEIGHT LOSS

Wall Pilates is not just about toning muscles, it's also a great way to shed unwanted pounds. By engaging and working your core muscles, Wall Pilates helps you burn more calories. This low-impact form of exercise also increases your heart rate without putting undue strain on your body, making it a safe and effective way to get a great workout. Plus, Wall Pilates can help you build muscle tone and definition in the arms, legs, and core, which helps create the calorie deficit needed for weight loss. With dedication and the right routine and diet, Wall Pilates can be a powerful tool to help you reach your weight loss goals and achieve a healthier, happier you.

IMPROVES BALANCE AND COORDINATION

Looking to enhance your coordination and balance? Wall Pilates might just be the solution you need! This type of Pilates challenges your body to use multiple muscles in a coordinated fashion, thereby improving your stability and balance. By incorporating wall Pilates into your fitness routine, you can increase your agility and mobility for everyday activities such as sports or walking. Furthermore, wall Pilates can also improve your reflexes, enabling you to respond promptly to unexpected situations. This is crucial not only for sports but also for day-to-day tasks like catching a falling object or avoiding hazards. With regular practice, wall Pilates can reduce the risk of falls and injuries while improving your overall balance and coordination. Give it a try today and experience the benefits for yourself!

GREAT STRESS RELIEVER

Looking to reduce stress levels? Wall Pilates can be a fantastic way to achieve this. By using the wall as support, you can enjoy a low-impact workout that's safe and effective. As you focus on controlled movement and breathing patterns, you can release tension and stress in your body. Furthermore, Wall Pilates can help improve your posture, which can also reduce stress and tension. As you breathe deeply and concentrate on your movements, you can experience a sense of calm and relaxation that can carry over into your daily life. The endorphins released during exercise can also contribute to an improved mood and reduced stress levels. So why not give Wall Pilates a try and see how it can help you manage stress and find inner peace?

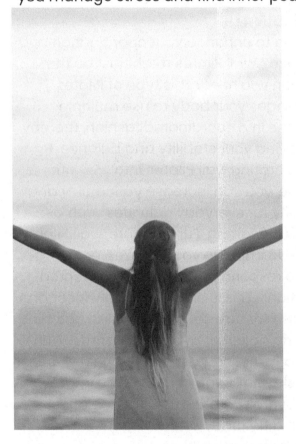

CAN HELP IMPROVE SLEEP

Wall Pilates can do wonders for improving sleep quality. Studies show that regular exercise can regulate body temperature, making it easier to fall asleep and stay asleep. In addition, Wall Pilates can help reduce stress and fatigue, which are common causes of insomnia. It also helps to relax the mind and body, allowing you to unwind before bed. Moreover, because Wall Pilates is a low-impact form of exercise, it won't interfere with your sleep if done before bedtime. So if you're looking for a way to improve your sleep, try incorporating Wall Pilates into your routine. With regular practice, you may notice an improvement in your sleep quality and overall well-being. Say goodbye to restless nights and hello to better sleep with Wall Pilates!

CAN HELP RELIEVE BACK PAIN

Back pain can be a debilitating issue that affects people of all ages and backgrounds. Fortunately, Wall Pilates provides a gentle, low-impact solution that can help alleviate back pain. This method strengthens your core muscles, improves your posture, and helps you move in a more mindful and controlled way.

When practicing Wall Pilates, you move slowly and deliberately while focusing on your breath, which can have a calming effect on both your mind and body. This mindful approach allows you to pinpoint areas of tension in your back and work to release it.

Moreover, the strengthening of your core muscles supports your spine and maintains proper posture, reducing pressure on your lower back. This leads to improved stability, flexibility, and balance, making everyday activities more comfortable and easier to do.

Wall Pilates also incorporates stretching, which is beneficial in increasing blood flow to your muscles, helping with recovery and realigning your vertebrae. Stretching also enhances your flexibility, which can alleviate stiffness and reduce back pain.

Overall, Wall Pilates is an effective and empowering way to reduce or eliminate back pain. By focusing on alignment, strength, and flexibility, Wall Pilates can provide relief from back pain and improve the quality of your life. Try it today and feel the difference it can make in your overall well-being.

REDUCES TIGHTNESS AND SORENESS IN MUSCLES

Wall Pilates is a powerful tool for reducing tension and soreness in the muscles. With its focus on controlled movements and deep breathing, Wall Pilates helps to engage all the major muscle groups in the body, promoting circulation and improving range of motion. As you practice Wall Pilates, you'll be able to stretch and release tension and soreness in your muscles, helping to reduce chronic pain and discomfort. Wall Pilates is a great way to improve flexibility, which can be incredibly beneficial in everyday life.

Whether you're reaching for something high on a shelf, bending down to tie your shoes, or simply walking up the stairs, having greater flexibility can make these activities easier and less uncomfortable. By practicing Wall Pilates regularly, you can also improve your overall sense of relaxation and well-being, helping to reduce stress and promote a greater sense of calm in your daily life.

REDUCES SORENESS IN JOINTS AND LIGAMENTS

Wall Pilates is a wonderful way to keep your joints and ligaments feeling flexible and healthy. With a unique blend of stretching and strengthening exercises, Pilates can help realign your body, reducing pressure and strain on your joints and ligaments. This means you can enjoy more ease of movement, and participate in your favorite activities without experiencing discomfort or pain. Plus, wall Pilates can help to prevent joint stiffness and weakness, which can lead to injury or decreased mobility over time. By practicing wall Pilates regularly, you can maintain the flexibility and health of your joints and ligaments, allowing you to feel strong, supple, and capable in your body.

INCREASES FLEXIBILITY

Wall Pilates is a practice that can transform your physical health and wellbeing. By focusing on increasing flexibility, Wall Pilates helps you become more agile and mobile, making daily activities easier and more comfortable. The combination of stretching and strengthening exercises can help you improve joint mobility and reduce the risk of injury by encouraging proper form and technique. With regular practice, you will begin to notice a significant increase in your range of motion, helping you to move more freely and without discomfort. Wall Pilates also provides a space for you to connect with your body, cultivating a sense of mindfulness and inner calm that can positively impact all areas of your life.

IMPROVES CONFIDENCE AND SELF-ESTEEM

Wall Pilates can do wonders for your confidence and self-esteem. By strengthening and toning your body, improving your posture, and increasing your balance and flexibility, wall Pilates can help you feel more comfortable and confident in your own skin. This confidence boost can extend beyond the walls of the studio, improving your overall outlook on life. Additionally, the focus and discipline required to master the wall Pilates moves can give you a sense of accomplishment and pride in your abilities, further boosting your self-esteem. With regular practice, wall Pilates can help you not only feel better physically, but also more confident and empowered in all aspects of your life.

BUILDS RESILIENCE

Resilience is a crucial quality for navigating life's challenges, and wall pilates can help you develop it. By building physical and mental strength, endurance, and flexibility, wall pilates helps you become more resilient. Regular practice can improve your ability to cope with stress and bounce back from difficult situations. The strengthening and stretching exercises of wall pilates can help you build up your physical endurance and resistance to fatigue, as well as improve your mental focus and concentration. As you become stronger and more flexible in your body and mind, you'll be better equipped to handle life's ups and downs with grace and resilience.

IMPROVES MOOD

With its unique combination of stretching, strengthening, and breathing exercises, Wall Pilates can be a powerful mood booster. The mind-body connection in Pilates helps to reduce stress and anxiety, leaving you feeling more relaxed and centered. Wall Pilates also improves blood flow, which can lead to increased energy levels and a greater sense of well-being. As you become more skilled in Wall Pilates, you may find that your mood improves, and you feel more positive and optimistic about life. And the best part is, you don't need any special equipment to do wall pilates, just a wall and your own body. Not only can Wall Pilates improve your mood, but it can also give you a sense of accomplishment and self-confidence as you progress and perfect your technique.

DEVELOPS MINDFULNESS

Mindfulness is the practice of being present in the moment and aware of your thoughts, feelings, and sensations. Wall Pilates helps you develop mindfulness by focusing on each movement and exercise, which allows you to become more aware of your body and how it moves. By staying focused on your breath and body alignment, you can improve your coordination and balance while reducing mental and physical stress. Practicing mindfulness through wall pilates can also help you gain a deeper understanding of your body and how it works, which can lead to greater self-awareness and a sense of calm. Ultimately, wall pilates is a holistic approach to wellness that can benefit both the mind and body.

IMPROVES INDEPENDENCE

Wall Pilates is a wonderful way for people to improve their physical and mental wellbeing. It offers a low-impact workout that is gentle on joints and muscles, making it an ideal exercise for those with limited mobility. As seniors age, their core muscles and balance can weaken, which can lead to a lack of confidence in their movement. By practicing wall Pilates, anybody at any age can strengthen their core muscles and improve balance, which can help them move with ease and confidence. This can result in increased independence and the ability to enjoy activities for seniors people. Wall Pilates can also improve flexibility and reduce stiffness in the body. It can also boost mood and reduce stress, contributing to an overall improved quality of life for seniors..

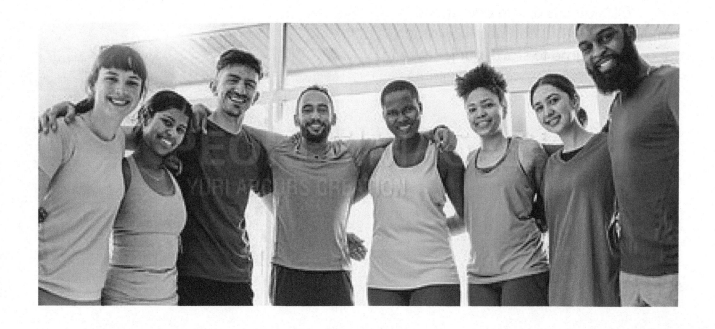

CAN AID IN PHYSICAL REHABILITATION

Wall Pilates is a form of exercise that can benefit those who are recovering from an injury or dealing with chronic pain.
This low-impact workout is gentle on the body and helps to build strength and flexibility while minimizing the risk of further injury. Wall Pilates can increase range of motion, reduce muscle soreness and stiffness, and help stabilize joints. It is particularly effective for improving balance and postural alignment, which are crucial for physical rehabilitation.
By focusing on specific muscle groups, Wall Pilates helps improve overall coordination and stability, which can reduce the risk of re-injury. With consistent practice, individuals can gain more confidence in their movements and improve their overall quality of life. Wall Pilates is also a great way to manage chronic pain and improve mobility, making it an ideal option for those who are recovering from an injury or surgery.
If you're looking to rebuild your strength, increase flexibility, and rehabilitate from an injury, Wall Pilates is a safe and effective form of exercise that can help you reach your goals. It's time to start your journey to recovery and wellness with Wall Pilates.

REDUCES DEPRESSION AND ANXIETY

Are you ready to feel a sense of calm and relaxation? Wall Pilates might just be the answer to your mental health needs. If you're struggling with anxiety or depression, the practice of wall pilates can help ease your mind and lift your mood. By focusing on your breath and each movement, you'll find yourself in the present moment, free from worries about the past or future. As you stretch your muscles and release tension, endorphins will flood your system, leaving you feeling happier and more energized. And the positive self-talk that comes with wall pilates can help you cultivate a kinder, more compassionate inner voice. So, if you're ready to let go of stress and negative emotions, give wall pilates a try and experience the transformative power of mindfulness and movement.

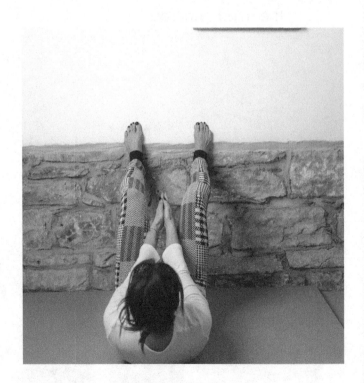

PRECAUTIONS

Wall Pilates provides numerous benefits for people of all ages, such as enhancing strength, flexibility, and balance. But just like any other form of exercise, it's crucial to be mindful of potential risks, particularly for seniors. In this chapter, we'll discuss the various potential hazards associated with Wall Pilates and provide practical tips to ensure safe practice. We'll delve into critical factors such as proper technique and recognizing your body's limitations. With our expert guidance, you'll be able to engage in Wall Pilates with confidence and stay healthy while reaping the many benefits this form of exercise has to offer.

IMPORTANCE OF WARMING UP

Let me tell you how crucial warming up is before practicing Wall Pilates! Not only does it prepare your body for the exercise, but it also reduces the risk of injury and helps you perform better. Warming up increases your heart rate and blood flow, which brings oxygen and nutrients to your muscles, preparing them for the workout ahead. It also loosens up your joints allowing you to move more freely during the practice. By taking the time to properly warm up, you're setting yourself up for success and maximizing the benefits of Wall Pilates. So, let's make sure to never skip the warm-up and give our bodies the attention and care they deserve!

FALLS

When it comes to Wall Pilates, safety should always be a top priority. While this form of exercise can be beneficial for people of all ages, it's crucial to understand the potential risks involved and take the necessary precautions to avoid injury.

One of the most important things to keep in mind is proper form. Incorrect technique can put unnecessary strain on your muscles and joints, leading to injury. It's essential to have a trained instructor guide you through the movements and make sure you're doing them correctly. Another risk to be aware of is overexertion. It can be tempting to push yourself to your limits in order to see results quickly, but this can lead to burnout and injury. It's important to start slowly and gradually increase the intensity of your workouts as your body becomes stronger and more comfortable with the exercises.

For seniors, it's especially important to take into account any pre-existing medical conditions or physical limitations. Certain movements may need to be modified or avoided altogether to prevent injury. It's also crucial to listen to your body and not push yourself beyond your limits. By staying mindful of potential risks and taking the necessary precautions, you can enjoy the many benefits of this form of exercise without putting your health at risk.

MUSCLE STRAINS

Muscle strains are no joke. They can happen to anyone, regardless of age, but they can be particularly dangerous for seniors who may not have the same level of flexibility as younger people. That's why it's so important to practice Wall Pilates exercises slowly and carefully, always taking breaks to allow your muscles to rest and recover. And remember, self-care is essential for long-term success in any fitness program.

Starting a new fitness program is always exciting, but it's important to remember that your body needs time and rest to adapt and recover. Overworking your muscles can lead to serious injury, which could ultimately set you back in your fitness journey. So, take care of yourself and give your body the care and attention it deserves.

But perhaps the most important thing to keep in mind is listening to your body cues. If you're feeling tired or in pain, don't push yourself to power through. Ignoring your body's signals could lead to further injury, and ultimately derail your fitness goals. So, be kind to yourself and work in partnership with your body, not against it. By taking care of yourself and listening to your body's needs, you can safely and successfully incorporate Wall Pilates into your fitness routine.

JOINT INJURIES

Wall Pilates can really transform your body and mind. However, it's important to remember that there are certain risks involved, especially when it comes to joint injuries. These injuries can occur from overstretching or not maintaining proper alignment during exercises.

To prevent joint injuries during Wall Pilates, it's essential to know your body's limitations and not push yourself too far beyond what you can handle. Listen to your body, and be aware of any discomfort or pain you may be feeling in your joints. Always maintain proper alignment during each exercise to ensure you're engaging the right muscles and preventing any potential joint pain or injury.

Remember, Wall Pilates is a journey, not a destination. So take your time and be patient with yourself. Don't rush the process or try to do too much too soon. And, most importantly, if you experience any pain or discomfort, stop immediately and seek professional medical advice. By taking these necessary precautions, you'll be able to fully enjoy the benefits of Wall Pilates without any worries or risks of joint injuries.

HEAT EXHAUSTION

When practicing wall Pilates, it is important to be aware of the potential dangers of heat exhaustion. The human body is vulnerable to the heat, especially during exercise. Heat exhaustion can occur when you overexert yourself in an environment that is too hot or humid. This can lead to symptoms such as excessive sweating, dizziness, confusion, and fatigue.

If you experience any of these symptoms while practicing wall Pilates, it is important to take a break immediately and move to a cooler area. Make sure to drink plenty of fluids and replace lost electrolytes. It is also important to wear appropriate clothing and to avoid exercising during the hottest part of the day.

We all know how tempting it is to push ourselves to the limit, but when it comes to heat exhaustion, there is no room for compromise. If you experience symptoms that persist, it is crucial to seek medical attention as soon as possible. By taking the necessary precautions and being mindful of your body's needs, you can enjoy the benefits of wall Pilates without putting yourself at risk of heat exhaustion.

DEHYDRATION

Wall Pilates can be a great form of exercise for seniors, but it is important to be aware of the dangers of heat exhaustion. This can happen when you overexert yourself in an environment that is too hot, or if you are wearing heavy clothing. Symptoms of heat exhaustion include excessive sweating, dizziness, confusion, and fatigue. If these symptoms occur, it is important to take a break and move to a cooler area. It is also important to drink plenty of fluids and replace electrolytes. If symptoms persist, it is important to seek medical attention immediately.

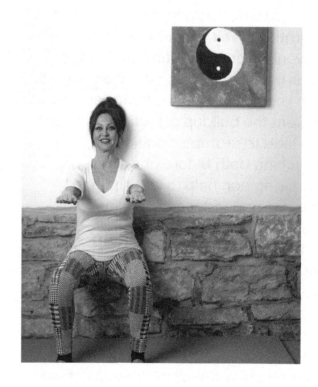

CRAMPS

t's always important to take extra precautions to avoid injury during exercise. One common issue that many seniors face is cramps during wall Pilates. These painful muscle contractions can be caused by overworking the muscles and not allowing them enough rest and recovery time. However, there are steps you can take to prevent cramps and keep your body feeling its best.

Firstly, be sure to take frequent breaks throughout your workout. This will give your muscles the chance to rest and prevent them from becoming overworked and tight. Using a foam roller can also help relax tight muscles and increase blood flow to the affected areas. Hydration is key when it comes to preventing cramps. Drinking plenty of fluids before and after your workout will help keep your muscles hydrated and prevent the buildup of lactic acid that can lead to cramps. Additionally, stretching both before and after exercising can help to loosen tight muscles and reduce the likelihood of experiencing cramps.

It's important to listen to your body and not push yourself too hard during exercise. If you feel any pain or discomfort, take a break and allow your body to recover. With the right precautions and a little bit of self-care, you can enjoy the many benefits of wall Pilates without the risk of cramps or injury. So, let's prioritize our health and take the necessary steps to prevent cramps and stay feeling our best.

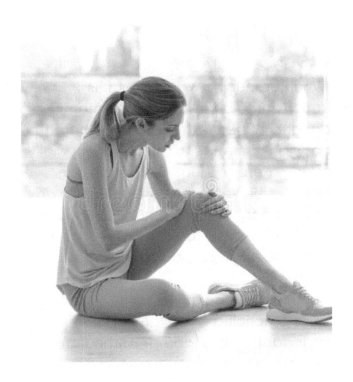

RHABDOMYOLYSIS

R Rhabdomyolysis is a rare but potentially life-threatening condition that can occur during exercise. This happens when muscle tissue breaks down, and the proteins and electrolytes released into the bloodstream.

To reduce the risk of rhabdomyolysis, it's important to take the necessary precautions before and after performing wall Pilates exercises. This includes properly warming up and cooling down, drinking plenty of fluids before, during, and after the workout, and not pushing yourself beyond your limits. It's also important to pay attention to your body and be aware of any signs of overexertion or muscle strain. Remember, your health and safety should always come first, so take the necessary steps to prevent any potential health complications.

IMPORTANCE OF BREATHING

it is crucial to maintain physical activity to stay healthy and strong. However, we must also be mindful of our bodies and take precautions to avoid injury. One way to do this during wall Pilates is by focusing on proper breathing technique. Proper breathing not only helps prevent injury but also improves the overall effectiveness of the workout. Seniors should pay close attention to their breath during exercise and avoid holding their breath or breathing too shallowly. In this blog post, we will delve into the benefits of proper breathing during wall Pilates for seniors and provide tips to ensure that you are breathing correctly during physical activity. By prioritizing proper breathing techniques, seniors can enjoy the benefits of wall Pilates while reducing the risk of injury.

WHAT IS PROPER BREATHING?

Proper breathing is not just a mere activity, it is an art that can transform our health and wellbeing. Seniors engaging in Wall Pilates and other exercises can benefit greatly from proper breathing techniques. It can help seniors maximize the benefits of exercise, minimize injury, and even enhance the mind-body connection.

By practicing proper breathing techniques, seniors can regulate their heart rate, improve digestion, and oxygenate their tissues and organs. Proper breathing also helps reduce stress and anxiety, which are common issues that seniors face. Moreover, it can improve sleep quality, which is essential for seniors to maintain their health. During Wall Pilates and other exercises, proper breathing techniques help increase the effectiveness of the activity. It ensures that the body is receiving enough oxygen and nutrients to strengthen and stretch the muscles. Proper breathing also enhances focus, coordination, and balance during the activity.

To practice proper breathing during Wall Pilates and other exercises, seniors should inhale deeply through the nose and exhale slowly through the mouth. This type of mindful breathing helps bring oxygen to the muscles and organs in order to promote physical and mental relaxation. It also helps prevent the body from becoming overly stressed or fatigued during exercise. By incorporating proper breathing techniques into their exercise routine, seniors can experience the full benefits of physical activity and maintain a healthy and active lifestyle.

THE DANGERS OF POOR BREATHING TECHNIQUES

It is important for everybody to practice proper breathing techniques when doing any type of exercise, especially wall Pilates. Poor breathing can be dangerous for people of all ages. For example, it can cause shallow breathing which leads to low oxygen levels in the body. This can then cause fatigue and an increased heart rate, both of which can be dangerous. Additionally, improper breathing can cause hyperventilation and dizziness, which can also lead to accidents.

For these reasons, it is important for everyone to practice proper breathing techniques when engaging in any type of exercise. Not only will proper breathing help to avoid the aforementioned dangers, it will also help individuals achieve maximum benefit from their workouts. Proper breathing helps to increase oxygen levels in the body, improve endurance and increase circulation. All of these things can be beneficial for individuals as th

Finally proper breathing helps to increase oxygen levels in the body, improve endurance and increase circulation. All of these things can be beneficial for seniors as they engage in exercise.

THE BENEFITS OF PROPER BREATHING

Discover the transformative power of proper breathing during Wall Pilates and other exercises! By practicing correct breathing techniques, everybody can reap a multitude of health benefits. Not only can it maintain a healthy heart rate and reduce stress and anxiety, but it can also improve energy levels and mood. Furthermore, proper breathing can help maintain optimal blood pressure and oxygen levels, enabling the body to work more efficiently, reduce fatigue, and improve performance during Wall Pilates and other exercises. Proper breathing techniques can also help to increase the range of motion in joints, promoting better balance and coordination. Whether dealing with arthritis or back pain due to poor posture or aging, proper breathing can help alleviate pain and discomfort. Additionally, proper breathing techniques can help to calm the mind and body, promoting better sleep and reducing stress levels. Taking slow, deep breaths can have a profound effect on the nervous system, improving mental clarity and overall wellbeing. Don't underestimate the power of proper breathing - start incorporating it into your exercise routine today!

TIPS FOR PROPER BREATHING WHILE DOING PILATES

CONCENTRATE ON YOUR BREATHING
Preparing for a Pilates exercise requires focusing on your breath. Take a few moments to inhale and exhale deeply, allowing your body to relax and concentrate on your breath. This will help you set the right tone for your practice.

PRACTICE RHYTHMIC BREATHING
Breathe with intention during your Pilates workout and keep your inhalations and exhalations in a steady rhythm. This will not only help you maintain control over your movements but also connect your body and mind for a more effective workout.

COORDINATE WITH MOVEMENTS
WAs you engage in Pilates exercises, strive to synchronize your breath with your movements. Take a deep inhale before initiating the exercise and exhale as you perform the movement. This allows for a more effective and efficient workout that can enhance your overall physical and mental well-being.

KEEP YOUR CORE ENGAGED
During your Pilates routine, engage your core muscles by gently contracting your abdominal muscles and lifting up through your ribcage, while keeping your shoulders relaxed and down. This will help you maintain good posture, prevent hunching or slouching, and facilitate proper breathing throughout your workout.

BE MINDFUL
When you're doing Pilates, it's important to be aware of your breath. Don't rush through exercises or forget to breathe altogether. Listen to your body and don't forget to take breaks if you need them.

By following these tips, you can make sure that you're properly breathing while doing Pilates exercises. Proper breathing is an essential part of staying safe and maximizing the benefits of Pilates for seniors. With practice and dedication, you can soon be reaping the rewards of proper breathing and enjoying all the benefits Pilates has to offer.

YOUR COMMITMENT IS IMPORTANT

Embarking on a journey to improve your health and wellness requires commitment and motivation to achieve your desired goals. With our 28-day Wall Pilates program, we believe in tailoring exercises and personalized instruction to help you learn proper technique and optimize the effectiveness of your movements.

Wall Pilates can make a world of difference in staying committed to your health and wellness goals. Our simple routines provide step-by-step instructions and detailed pictures of each exercise to guide you through the process. You can even invite your partner or a friend to join in for a little friendly competition - it's always satisfying to be stronger than your other half, no matter your age.

In addition to guidance and support, Wall Pilates provides accountability to keep you consistently moving forward towards your goals. This is especially important when you're struggling to stay motivated and on track. Having a consistent plan of action and accountability to complete it can help you overcome challenges and push through even the toughest times.

Finally, committing to yourself and Wall Pilates allows you to celebrate your progress and accomplishments. Celebrating small successes along the way is important in developing healthy habits and maintaining motivation. With Wall Pilates, you'll have access to performance tracking to recognize when you're making progress and gaining strength, as well as when you need to adjust your routine to keep progressing. By making a commitment to yourself and Wall Pilates, you're taking control of your health and well-being and arming yourself with the best tools to achieve your goals. We believe in your potential to succeed and look forward to joining you on this journey towards a healthier, happier you.

WHAT DO YOU NEED TO GET STARTED

Getting started couldn't be easier. Wall Pilates doesn't require any fancy equipment or a lot of space. That's what makes it so perfect. If you're a senior looking for an exercise program that can improve your strength and mobility, then Pilates is a great choice! This low-impact exercise system has become popular among people of all ages. Senior citizens who have started doing Pilates can expect improved core strength, improved balance, better posture, increased flexibility and improved coordination.

The great thing about Pilates is that it doesn't require any expensive equipment or fancy classes, which makes it accessible to anyone of all abilities. With our 28-day wall Pilates program, you're going to receive everything you need from instructional images to step-by step instructions. So, we take away the guess work. All you need is simple equipment to make you feel more comfortable and safe during movements. To get started, you will need the following:

- A Mat: Invest in a good quality mat. You'll be using it often and for long periods of time, so it's important to have something that's comfortable and durable.
- Exercise Clothes: Exercise clothes should be light, breathable, and stretchy. Sweatpants or leggings are great options.
- Comfortable Shoes: While Pilates can be done without shoes, investing in a comfortable pair of sneakers is highly recommended, especially if you will be doing Pilates on a regular basis.

If you want to get the most out of your Pilates sessions, make sure you take the time to warm up your muscles and joints before each session. Always be aware of your body, and listen to its feedback during and after the exercise. Make sure to work within your range of abilities, and don't overexert yourself. If you feel any discomfort, make sure to stop immediately. Finally, practice good breathing technique throughout your session to get the best results from each exercise. With proper practice, you can soon start seeing the benefits of Pilates.

PILATES MOVEMENTS

The transformative power of wall Pilates is truly amazing! This type of exercise can help you build strength, increase your independence, and feel more confident in your day-to-day activities. With wall Pilates, you'll be able to conquer any task that comes your way with ease.

One of the best things about wall Pilates is that it's accessible to everyone, whether you're a beginner or an experienced fitness enthusiast. The basic wall Pilates poses are simple but effective, involving pressing your body into the wall and pushing out against it to work your muscles. These poses, such as wall squats, push-ups, planks, and crunches, can help you build strength and tone your body in a low-impact way. As you become more comfortable with the basic poses, you can challenge yourself with more advanced wall Pilates exercises. These poses involve moving your body in relation to the wall and using it for support, such as the wall press, wall lunge, and hip extension. These poses will help you further improve your strength and flexibility.

But no matter what level you're at, proper form and alignment are crucial in wall Pilates. By focusing on engaging your core muscles and maintaining proper posture, you can avoid injuries and get the most out of your workout. With good form, you can enjoy improved posture, better balance, and increased flexibility.

To ensure proper form while doing wall Pilates poses, it's important to pay attention to your body and make adjustments as needed. Remember to keep your core engaged, your spine straight, and your hips neutral. And don't forget to breathe deeply and evenly throughout your movements.

In conclusion, wall Pilates is an amazing exercise program that can help you build strength, increase your independence, and feel more confident in your daily activities. Whether you're a beginner or an experienced fitness enthusiast, this program is accessible to all. By focusing on proper form and alignment, you can enjoy the full benefits of wall Pilates and take your fitness to the next level!

BODY ALIGNMENT

Welcome to the chapter on body alignment in Pilates! This is where you'll learn the essential principles of proper body positioning during Pilates exercises. By mastering these fundamentals, you'll be able to fully maximize the benefits of your Pilates practice while minimizing the risk of injury. Let's dive in and start exploring!

WHAT IS BODY ALIGNMENT?

Welcome to the chapter that's all about body alignment during Pilates! Proper alignment is crucial to ensure that you get the most out of your Pilates practice while also minimizing the risk of injury. By focusing on the alignment of your body, shoulder blades, spine, pelvis, hip joints, knees, and ankles, you can create a solid foundation for your Pilates movements.

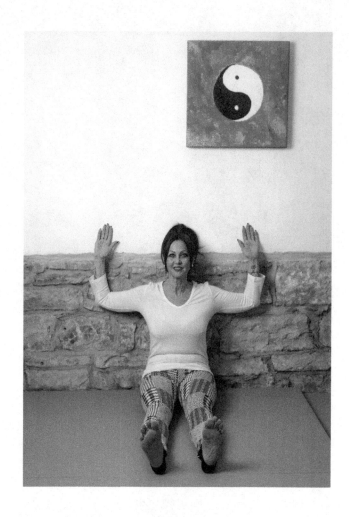

When it comes to alignment, it's all about creating straight lines between these points of the body. This means that your shoulder blades should be drawn down and away from your ears, your spine should be long and straight, your pelvis should be in a neutral position, your hip joints should be level and square, your knees should be in line with your feet, and your ankles should be strong and stable.

It's important to note that proper alignment isn't just about the physical positioning of your body; it's also about finding balance and equal weight distribution on both feet. By standing in a neutral position with your head directly over your spine, you can create a strong foundation for your Pilates practice and prevent unnecessary strain or injury. So let's focus on alignment and take our Pilates practice to the next level!

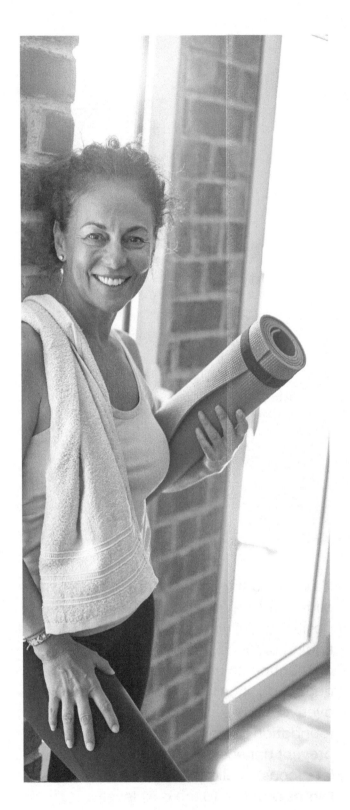

Body alignment will help activate the deep core muscles that are essential for stability and support.

Another key element of body alignment is maintaining proper posture in all positions. When standing, make sure that your weight is evenly distributed on both feet and that your knees are in line with your ankles. Keep your shoulders back and down, and imagine that you have a string pulling you up from the top of your head.

When lying down, make sure that your entire spine is in contact with the mat, and that your head and neck are in a neutral position. Your shoulder blades should be relaxed and your arms should be at your sides.

By following these basic principles of body alignment, you can ensure that you get the most out of your Pilates practice. Not only will you improve your posture and core strength, but you will also reduce your risk of injury and increase your overall wellbeing.

Get ready to feel the burn and strengthen your core with Wall Pilates! By engaging your core muscles and supporting your spine throughout the workout, you'll be able to take your practice to the next level.

Don't forget to maintain a neutral pelvic position to ensure proper balance and muscle activation. It's essential to practice good body alignment in order to get the maximum benefit from each move and reduce the risk of injury.

With dedication and focus, you'll be able to perfect your form and achieve amazing results in your Pilates practice. So, let's get started and unleash the power of Wall Pilates!

DANGERS OF POOR BODY ALIGNMENT DURING PILATES

Having the proper body alignment during Pilates is essential to avoid a range of issues, such as injuries, joint pains, and overworking of certain muscles.

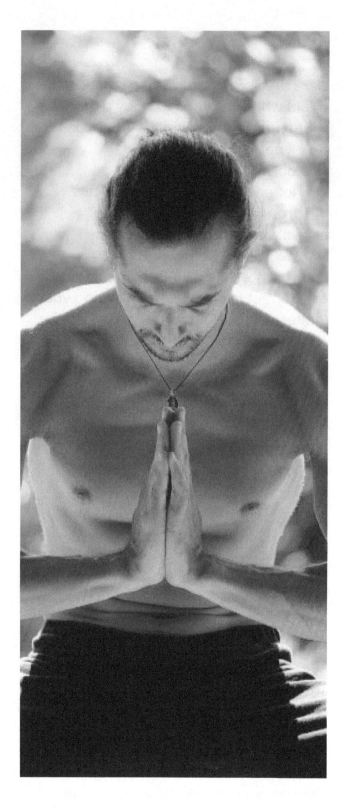

Poor body alignment can lead to decreased posture, flexibility, and stability, which can affect the efficiency of your Pilates practice. By focusing on maintaining proper alignment and engaging your core muscles, you can prevent these issues and ensure that you get the most out of your Pilates workouts.

Remember, taking care of your body through proper alignment is crucial for achieving a fulfilling and rewarding Pilates practice.

Here are some common mistakes to avoid when it comes to body alignment:

- Bending or arching the back too far
- Hyper-extending joints
- Locking out joints
- Not engaging the core muscles properly
- Not using the breath properly

If you're not sure if you're maintaining the correct body alignment during your Pilates practice, it's important to ask for help from a trained professional. They can help ensure that you're performing each exercise correctly and safely, while still getting the most out of your practice.

TIPS FOR IMPROVING YOUR BODY ALIGNMENT

START WITH A STRONG FOUNDATION

To get the most out of your Pilates practice, it's crucial to start with a solid foundation. This means beginning your session by focusing on your body's base - your feet. Take the time to ensure that your feet are firmly rooted on the ground, and then work your way up, checking that your ankles, hips, and shoulders are all in perfect alignment. With a strong foundation, you'll be able to perform your Pilates exercises with greater ease, stability, and precision, allowing you to achieve your fitness goals in no time!

ENGAGE YOUR CORE MUSCLES

Pay close attention to your core muscles and keep them engaged throughout the session. This will help ensure your body is properly aligned and will also increase the intensity of your workout.

DON'T FORGET TO BREATHE

Breathing is a powerful tool to maintain proper body alignment during Pilates. Take deep breaths that expand your lungs and push out your belly as you inhale, then release your abdominal muscles as you exhale. This will help you stay focused and centered throughout your practice.

KEEP YOUR HEAD IN LINE

Your head position plays a vital role in maintaining proper body alignment during Pilates. Keep your neck elongated, your shoulders relaxed and avoid jutting your chin forward. By maintaining the right head posture, you can enhance the benefits of your Pilates exercises and protect yourself from any potential injuries.

BE MINDFUL OF POSTURE

Maximizing your Pilates practice requires paying attention to your body's alignment from head to toe. Focus on maintaining a long, lifted spine, engaged core muscles, and relaxed shoulders throughout each exercise. Keep your neck in line with your spine, avoid arching or rounding in the lower back, and take deep breaths to promote good alignment

THE IMPORTANCE OF CONTROL

One of the key elements of a successful Pilates practice is the use of controlled movements. In this chapter, you'll discover how to use controlled movements to achieve better results in your Pilates practice. You'll learn how to engage your muscles properly and move with purpose, reducing the risk of injury and maximizing the effectiveness of each exercise. With detailed instructions and helpful tips, you'll be able to master the art of controlled movements .

WHY IS IT SO IMPORTANT?

My Pilates journey has taught me the importance of executing controlled movements. When movements are done with control, it ensures that all the muscles in the body are being worked, and not just a select few. It also helps to engage the deeper muscles, which can provide more stability and protection for the joints and spine. I have found that controlled movements have improved my coordination, balance, and alignment, which are all key components of Pilates. Additionally, executing controlled movements has helped me to develop a stronger mind-body connection and allowed me to get the most out of my practice.

In summary, controlled movements are essential to getting the most out of a Pilates practice, and I recommend incorporating them into your routine to see the benefits for yourself.

HOW TO EXECUTE CONTROLLED MOVEMENTS

One of the key components of Pilates is executing controlled movements. Control is essential for proper alignment and form, which are vital to prevent injury and maximize effectiveness. Here are some tips for executing controlled movements during a Pilates workout:

FOCUS ON YOUR BREATH

As you flow through each Pilates exercise, let your breath guide you. Inhale and exhale with intention, moving in a slow and steady rhythm to keep your body relaxed and your form on point.

ENGAGE YOUR CORE

It is important to ensure that your core muscles are activated while performing each exercise. This will ensure that you maintain proper alignment and stability, ultimately leading to more efficient movements.

KEEP IT SLOW AND DELIBERATE
Take your time with each exercise and move deliberately to maintain proper form and prevent injury.

PAY ATTENTION TO YOUR FORM
Maintain proper form throughout every exercise by checking your posture regularly and making necessary adjustments for optimal results.

USE PROPS
Enhance your Pilates practice with the use of props like yoga blocks, straps, or balls to improve alignment and control.

Maximize the benefits of Pilates with controlled movements. Follow these tips for better form and improved control, leading to better results with regular practice.

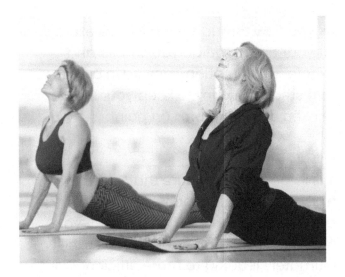

EXERCISES TO TRY TO PRACTICE CONTROL
When it comes to practicing control in Pilates, there are a few specific exercises that can help you to achieve this. Here's a few to try:

WALL SUPPORTED SQUAT
he Wall Supported Squat is a simple yet effective lower body exercise that helps strengthen the quads, hamstrings, and glutes. To perform this exercise, stand with your back against a wall, with your feet shoulder-width apart. Slowly lower your body down into a squat position, while keeping your back against the wall. Hold the position for a few seconds before returning to the starting position. This exercise is great for beginners or those recovering from injury, as it provides added support and stability.

STANDING SIDE KICK
Standing Side Kick is a Pilates exercise that targets the hip abductors, or outer thighs. To perform this exercise, stand with your feet hip-width apart and lift one leg out to the side, keeping it straight. As you lift your leg, engage your glutes and outer thigh muscles to maintain stability. Lower your leg back down to the starting position and repeat on the other side. The Standing Side Kick can help improve hip stability, balance, and overall lower body strength.

STANCE CHANGING SQUAT

The stance changing squat is a variation of the traditional squat that challenges your balance, stability, and leg strength. Starting with your feet together, you step out into a wide stance, then perform a squat with proper form, and return to the starting position. This exercise targets the muscles in your legs, glutes, and core, while also improving your coordination and balance. The stance changing squat can be modified to increase or decrease the intensity, making it suitable for a variety of fitness levels.

CHEST WALL PUSH UPS

Chest wall push-ups are a bodyweight exercise that targets the chest, shoulders, and triceps. This exercise is performed by standing a few feet away from a wall and placing your palms on the wall, shoulder-width apart. Slowly bend your elbows and lower your chest towards the wall, keeping your body straight. Then, push yourself back to the starting position by extending your arms. This exercise is great for building upper body strength and can be modified to make it easier or harder depending on your fitness level.

"You are never too old to make fitness a part of your life - no matter your age, movement is the key to longevity and happiness."

THE WALL PILATES PROGRAM AND THE 28 DAYS CHALLENGE

Our wall Pilates program is very flexible and allows you to build on strength at your own pace. You don't have to perform advanced poses straight away to feel results. It's all about you and your current level. Be patient and be committed. Start with the daily tonic routine, and if you feel good, then move on to the next stage (and so on). Take your time and remember what we discussed throughout this book.

To begin, depending on how you're feeling, start with one routine a week and then performing the following routines the weeks after. Increase how often you're performing then with a goal in mind to train for 28 days (1 routine a week x 4 weeks)

So, it's all about building your strength gradually and helping you build enough strength that you can train for 28 days without pain or strain. In addition to building up your resilience, remember to stop 15-20 seconds between each exercise to give yourself time to rest. Overworking yourself can be bad for your heart, so make sure to do each routine at your own pace.

WARM UP AND COOL DOWN

Lastly, before we dive into the poses and exercises. It's important that you warm up and cool down before and after each routine. Doing this before and after exercise is an important part of any exercise routine. It helps increase range of motion in your muscles, improves your overall flexibility, and reduces your risk of injury. Additionally, stretching helps to relax and reduce muscle tension, so that your body is better able to perform during exercise and recover afterward.

Before beginning any workout challenge, make sure to remember about a warm up and cool down which can help to prepare your muscles for the activity to come. A short stretching routine can help increase blood flow to your muscles, and helps increase flexibility and range of motion. This means that when you do exercise, you'll be able to work with a wider range of motion and a greater range of motion. Additionally, when you warm up before a workout, you can help reduce any muscle soreness and help prepare your body for the exercise you're about to do.

Warm up exercises should always precede any physical activity, even light walking. These warm up exercises can be as simple as:

ARM CIRCLES
Make small circles with your arms and then switch to making large circles. Repeat 5 times in each direction.

TRUNK ROTATIONS
While sitting, slowly rotate your upper body from left to right. Repeat 10 times.

SHOULDER ROLLS
With arms straight and parallel to the ground, rotate your shoulders in small circles, forward and backward. Repeat 10 times.

After physical activity, cool down exercises help reduce soreness and reduce risk of injury. Cool down exercises should be done at a slow and steady pace, and can include:

SLOW WALKING
Walk at a slow and comfortable pace to help cool your muscles down and return to normal breathing and heart rate.

LEG STRETCHES
Stand up, hold onto a stable surface, and gently stretch your legs one at a time for about 10 seconds each.

CHAIR SIT:
Sit on the edge of a chair with good posture and your feet flat on the ground. Make sure your hips, knees and ankles are at 90 degree angles and hold for 15-30 seconds.

Warm up and cool down exercises should be done regularly, preferably once or twice a day. It's a good idea to start and end the day with simple stretching, walking or strengthening exercises to help keep your body flexible and prevent strain or injury. By taking a few minutes every day to do warm up and cool down exercises, seniors can maintain physical health and increase quality of life.

WALL PILATES ROUTINES

DAILY TONIC ROUTINE (10 MINS)

- Stance Changing Squat
- Seated Thoracic Rotation
- Seated Side Bends
- Seated Arm Mobility
- Alternating Pike Leg Lift
- Shoulder Circle (Right)
- Shoulder Circle (Left)
- Wall Supported Reverse Crunch
- RAlternative Wall Sit Calf Raises

FULL BODY SCUPLT ROUTINE (10 MINS)

- Wall Supported Lateral Squats
- SWall Supported Knee Raise
- Wall Angels
- Elevated Glute Bridge + Clamshell
- Wall Shoulder Taps
- KReach Through Crunch
- RStanding side kick (right)
- Standing side kick (left)
- Kneeling Windshield Whippers

BUTT SCULPT ROUTINE (14 MINS)

- Wall Supported Squat + Kickback.
- Standing Clamshells
- Single Leg Glute Bridge (Left)
- Single Leg Glute Bridge (Right)
- Wall Supported Lateral
- Fire Hydrant (Right)
- Fire Hydrant (Left)
- Stance Changing Squat
- Elevated Glute Bridge + Clamshell
- Dynamic Hip Flexor Stretch (left)
- Dynamic Hip Flexor Stretch (Right)
- Stance Changing Squat
- Wall Sit with Leg Extension
- Elevated Glute Bridge + Clamshell
- Dynamic Hip Flexor Stretch (Left)
- Dynamic Hip Flexor Stretch (Right)

ULTIMATE WALL ROUTINE (14 MINS)

- Dynamic Backward Lunge (Right)
- Dynamic Backward Lunge (Left)
- Elevated Glute Bridge
- Wall Shoulder Taps
- Wall sit Calf Raises
- Chest wall Push Ups
- Abdominal Twist
- Standing Side Kick (Right)
- Standing Side Kick (Left)
- Wall Push Up Plank
- Calf Raised Squat
- Wall Supported Bicycle Crunch
- LSingle Leg Glute Bridge (Left)
- Single Leg Glute Bridge (Right).

EXERCISE INSTRUCTIONS

STANCE CHANGING SQUAT (60 SEC)

This exercise stretches your hamstrings and calve muscles. It will mobilize your lower and upper back.

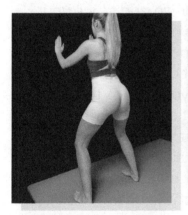
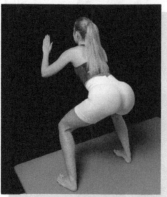
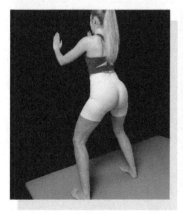
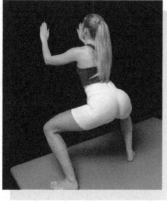

INSTRUCTIONS:

1. Stand a little bit away from the wall.
2. Put your hands on the wall
3. Take a bit wider stance
4. Squat down, and as you are coming up rotate your feet and
5. knees outwards
6. Squat down again and return to previous position.

COMMON MISTAKES TO AVOID

- Arching your back
- Holding the breath
- Rushing the movement

GENERAL TIPS:

- Inhale at the top of the movement, and exhale as you are ending the squat.

SEATED THORACIC ROTATION (60 SEC)

This exercise is a great way to work on your abdominal muscles while improving your thoracic spine mobility.

.

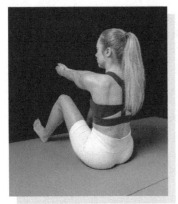 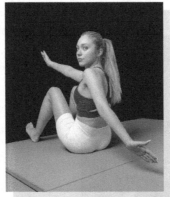

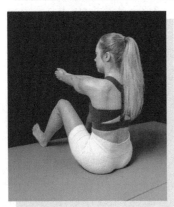 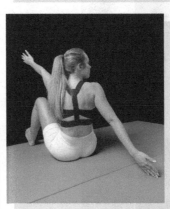

INSTRUCTIONS:

1. Sit down and place your toes against the wall.
2. Keep your knees slightly bent and lean back a bit.
3. Put your hands together in front of you.
4. Twist your arm and body to one side and touch the floor behind you.
5. Alternate between sides.

COMMON MISTAKES TO AVOID

- Rushing the movement.
- Holding your breath.
- Bending your spine.

GENERAL TIPS:

- Keep your core engaged throughout the exercise to reduce stress on your lower back.
- Move slowly and deliberately to ensure proper form and maximum benefit.

SEATED SIDE BENDS (60 SEC)

Seated Side Bends are a great exercise to work on your oblique muscles and improve spinal flexibility.

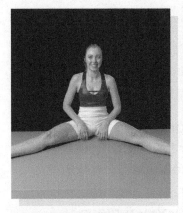
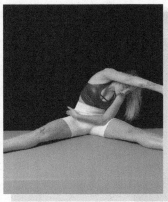
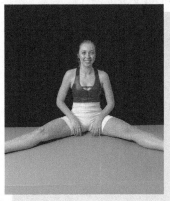
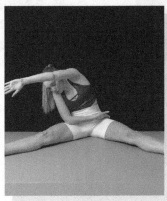

INSTRUCTIONS:

1. Sit tall to the the wall.
2. Put your back against the wall.
3. Straddle your Legs
4. Bend Your body to your left side while crossing your right arm over your head, reaching towards your toes.
5. Mirror the movement on the other side.

COMMON MISTAKES TO AVOID

- Rushing the movement.
- Holding your breath.
- Bending your legs and arm.

GENERAL TIPS:

- Keep your core engaged throughout the movement.
- Exhale as you bend to the side, inhale as you return to the starting position.

ALTERNATING PIKE LEG LIFT (60 SEC)

This exercise is a great way to challenge your hip flexors and improve your core strength.

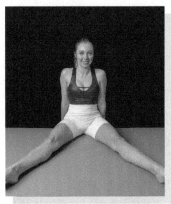 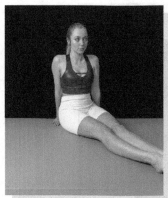

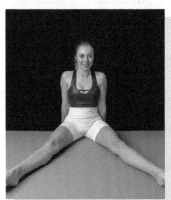 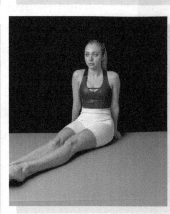

INSTRUCTIONS:

1. Sit tall against the wall with your legs straddled.
2. Place your hands on the floor.
3. Keeping your legs extended, lift your left leg up and bring.
4. Lower your left leg and repeat on the other side.
5. Alternate between legs.

COMMON MISTAKES TO AVOID

- Going too fast: Perform the movement slowly and with control.
- Holding your breath bending your legs

GENERAL TIPS:

- Maintain a regular breathing pattern while performing this exercise.
- Keep your legs as straight as possible to maximize the effectiveness of the exercise.

WALL SIT HIP HINGE (60 SEC)

Wall Sit Hip Hinge will stretch your hamstrings and glutes, and it will work onto your leg muscles. Your quadriceps tendons will also get stronger from this exercise.

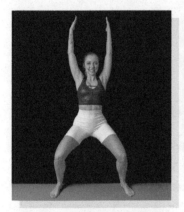
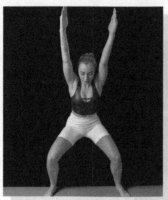
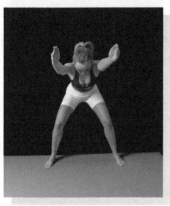

INSTRUCTIONS:

1. Put your back against the wall.
2. Keep your arms extended on the wall above your head.
3. Squat down until your knees are bent at a 90-degree angle.
4. From this position, lean forward until your chest is parallel to the floor.
5. slowly return to starting position.

COMMON MISTAKES TO AVOID

- Rushing the movement.
- Letting your glutes move away from the wall.
- Holding your breath.

GENERAL TIPS:

- Inhale at the top of the movement, and exhale as you start leaning your body forward.

SHOULDER CIRCLE (RIGHT) (60 SEC)

This exercise is great for improving shoulder mobility and can also be used as a warm-up exercise.

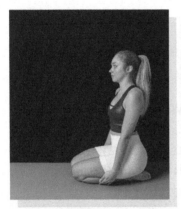
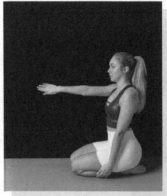

INSTRUCTIONS:

1. Kneel sideways of the wall and sit on your heels.
2. Place your hands onto your thighs
3. Make a circle with your right arm by combing your fingers over the wall.
4. While rotating your right arm look to your left side.

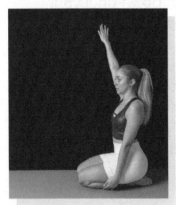
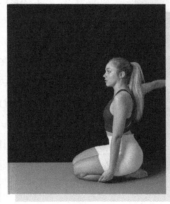

COMMON MISTAKES TO AVOID

- Rushing the movement.
- Holding your breath during the movement
- Arching your spine during the exercise.

GENERAL TIPS:

- Focus on the movement of your shoulder and avoid any unnecessary movement in your spine.
- Gradually increase the size of the circle as you feel more comfortable with the exercise.

SHOULDER CIRCLE (LEFT) (60 SEC)

This exercise is great for improving shoulder mobility and can also be used as a warm-up exercise.

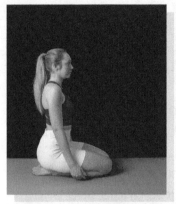
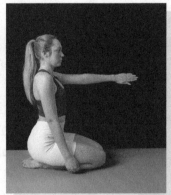
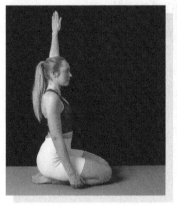
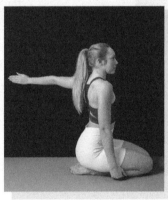

INSTRUCTIONS:

1. Kneel to the right side of a wall and sit on your heels.
2. Place your hands on your thighs.
3. Comb your fingers over the wall with your left arm to make a circle.
4. Return your leg to the starting position.
5. While rotating your left arm look towards your right side.

COMMON MISTAKES TO AVOID

- Rushing the movement.
- Holding your breath during the movement
- Arching your spine during the exercise.

GENERAL TIPS:

- Focus on the movement of your shoulder and avoid any unnecessary movement in your spine.
- Gradually increase the size of the circle as you feel more comfortable with the exercise.

WALL-SUPPORTED REVERSE CRUNCH (60 SEC)

This exercise is one of the best for strengthening your lower abdominal muscles.

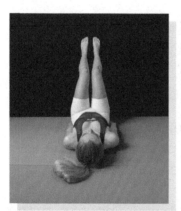
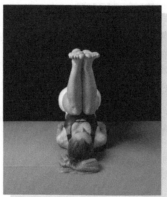
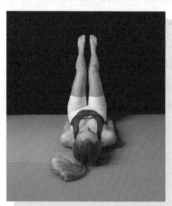

INSTRUCTIONS:

1. Lie on the floor with your feet together against the wall.
2. Bend your knees at a 90-degree angle and bring them together.
3. Lift your knees towards your chest and simultaneously raise your lower back off the floor.

COMMON MISTAKES TO AVOID

- Holding your breath.
- 1.Not allowing your lower back to move off the floor.
- Rushing the movement.

GENERAL TIPS:

- Inhale at the beginning of the movement and exhale as you bring your knees towards your chest.
- Keep your movements slow and controlled.

ALTERNATING WALL SIT CALF RAISES (90 SEC)

This exercise is great for improving your calf and ankle strength, as well as challenging your quadriceps muscles.

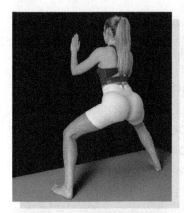
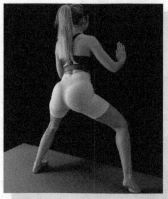
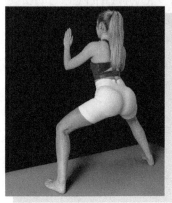
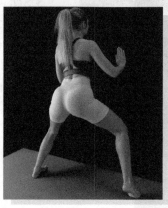

INSTRUCTIONS:

1. Stand tall facing the wall and place your hands on it.
2. Make your stance wide and slightly turn your feet outwards.
3. Squat down until your knees are at a 90-degree angle.
4. 1. Raise your left heel up, then lower it down and raise your right heel up.

COMMON MISTAKES TO AVOID

- Forgetting to alternate between the sides.
- Not squatting down to a 90-degree angle.

GENERAL TIPS:

- Maintain a regular breathing pattern while performing this exercise.
- Focus on performing the exercise with control and without rushing through the motion.

WALL SUPPORTED LATERAL SQUAT (60 SEC)

Wall Supported Lateral Squats. strengthens the quadriceps and glute muscles.

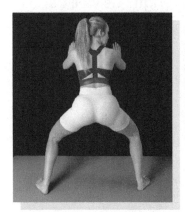 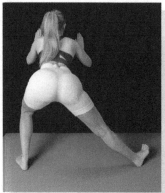

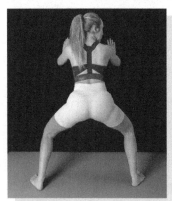 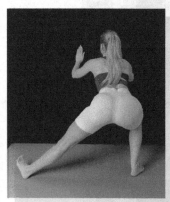

INSTRUCTIONS:

1. Stand facing a wall with your hands on it for support.
2. Keep your feet wider than hip-width apart and turn your toes out slightly.
3. Squat down and do a pulse squat on your right leg, while keeping your left leg extended to the side.
4. Alternate between legs.

COMMON MISTAKES TO AVOID

- Holding your breath.
- Rushing the movement.
- Not alternating between sides.

GENERAL TIPS:

- Inhale at the top of the movement.
- Exhale as you end the squat.

WALL SUPPORTED KNEE RAISE (60 SEC)

Wall Supported Knee Raise is a great exercise to activate your hip flexor and lower abdominal muscles.

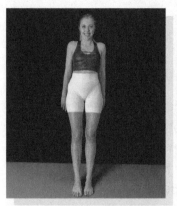
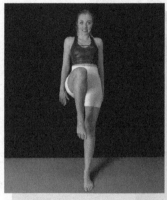
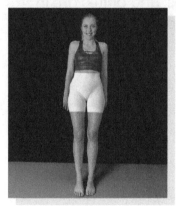
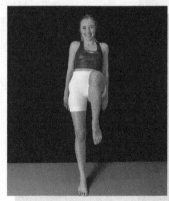

INSTRUCTIONS:

1. Lean your upper back against the wall.
2. Place your feet forward and keep them together.
3. Keep your arms and hands on the wall for support.
4. Lift your left knee up towards your chest.
5. Alternate between knees.

COMMON MISTAKES TO AVOID

- Not alternating between legs.
- Holding your breath.
- Not keeping contact with the wall

GENERAL TIPS:

- Keep your core engaged throughout the movement to help stabilize your body.
- Focus on lifting your knee up towards your chest, rather than just swinging it up.

WALL ANGELS (90 SEC)

Wall Angels are an excellent exercise that can improve your shoulder mobility and strengthen your upper back muscles.

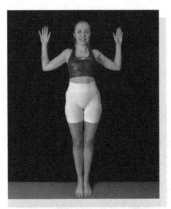
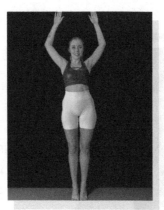
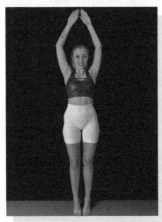

INSTRUCTIONS:

1. Stand tall with your feet together.
2. Extend your arms above your head and ensure that your upper back, forearms, wrists, and glutes are in contact with the wall.
3. Lift your heels up and slide your elbows down to a 45-degree angle.

COMMON MISTAKES TO AVOID

- Rushing through the movement.
- Losing contact with the wall.
- Holding your breath.

GENERAL TIPS:

- Inhale at the start of the movement and exhale slowly as you lift your heels.
- Perform the exercise slowly and with control to ensure proper form and engagement of the targeted muscles

ELEVATED GLUTE BRIDGE + CLAM SHELL (60 SEC)

This is a fantastic exercise that targets your glutes and hamstrings.

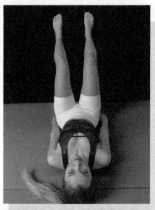
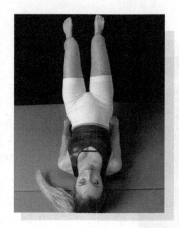
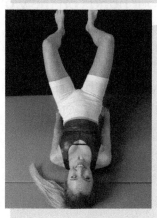

INSTRUCTIONS:

1. Lie on your back with your feet on the wall and your knees bent at a 90-degree angle.
2. Place your feet slightly higher than your knees.
3. Raise your hips up into a glute bridge position.
4. While keeping your hips lifted, open your knees to the side, then close them again.

COMMON MISTAKES TO AVOID

- Arching your back too much.
- Rushing the movement.
- Holding your breath.

GENERAL TIPS:

- Exhale as you open your knees and inhale as you close them.
- Focus on keeping your core engaged and your back flat on the ground.

WALL SHOULDER TAPS (60 SEC)

Wall Shoulder Taps are a great exercise that will improve your shoulder stability with minimal effort on the whole body.

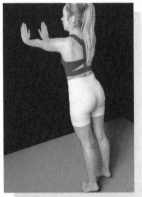 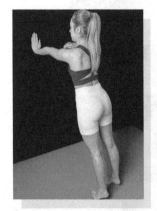

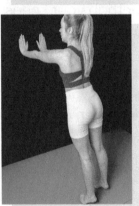 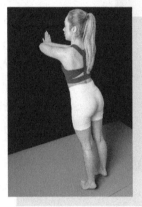

INSTRUCTIONS:

1. Stand tall a step or two away from the wall, while facing it.
2. Put your hands on the wall at your shoulder level.
3. Keep your feet together.
4. Touch your right shoulder with your left hand.
5. Alternate between sides.

COMMON MISTAKES TO AVOID

- Not alternating between sides
- Holding your breath
- Arching your spine
- Not keeping your core engaged

GENERAL TIPS:

- Maintain a regular breathing pattern while performing this exercise. Ensure that your core is engaged throughout the movement.

REACH THROUGH CRUNCH (60 SEC)

Reach Through Crunch is an excellent exercise that targets your abdominal muscles.

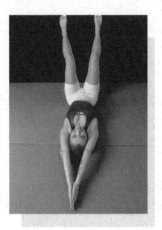 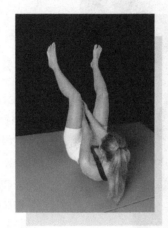

INSTRUCTIONS:

1. Lie flat on your back with your knees bent at a 90-degree angle and your feet on the floor.
2. Raise your arms over your head and bring your hands together.
3. Engage your core muscles and lift your shoulders off the floor.
4. Reach your hands between your knees and towards the wall behind you.
5. Return to the starting position and repeat.

COMMON MISTAKES TO AVOID

- Arching your lower back
- Failing to lift your shoulders off the floor
- Using momentum instead of controlled movement

GENERAL TIPS:

- Inhale as you lower your shoulders to the starting position and exhale as you crunch up.
- To increase the difficulty, try holding a lightweight or medicine ball in your hands during the exercise.

STANDING SIDE KICK (RIGHT) (60 SEC)

standing side kick is an exercise that targets can activates your glutes muscles and help build strength in that area.

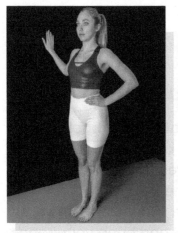 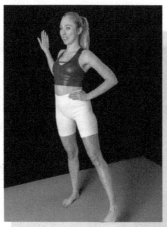

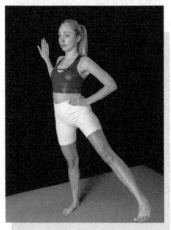

INSTRUCTIONS:

1. Stand sideways to the wall with your left hand on the wall and right hand on your hip.
2. Keep your feet together.
3. Without bending your body, kick sideways with your right leg.

COMMON MISTAKES TO AVOID

- Bending your knees.
- Allowing your body to bend while kicking sideways.
- Holding your breath.

GENERAL TIPS:

- Keep your core engaged and avoid leaning to the opposite side.
- Focus on lifting your leg with control, rather than swinging it.

STANDING SIDE KICK (LEFT) (60 SEC)

standing side kick is an exercise that targets can activates your glutes muscles and help build strength in that area.

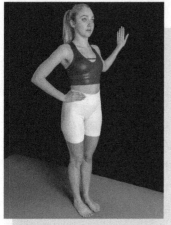
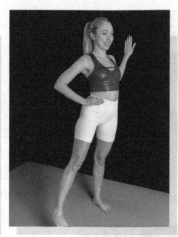
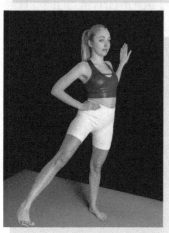

INSTRUCTIONS:

1. Stand sideways to the wall with your right hand on the wall and left hand on your hip.
2. Keep your feet together.
3. Without bending your body, kick sideways with your left leg.

COMMON MISTAKES TO AVOID

- Bending your knees.
- Allowing your body to bend while kicking sideways.
- Holding your breath.

GENERAL TIPS:

- Keep your core engaged and avoid leaning to the opposite side.
- Focus on lifting your leg with control, rather than swinging it.

KNEELING WINDSHIELD WIPERS (60 SEC)

Kneeling Windshield Wipers are an effective exercise that can mobilize and activate your lower back muscles while also engaging your core.

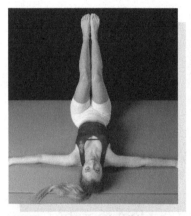
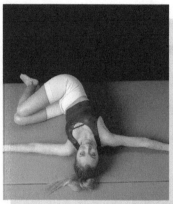
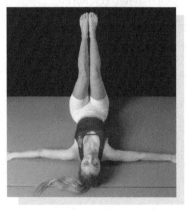
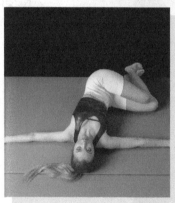

INSTRUCTIONS:

1. Start by lying on your back with your knees and feet together and propped up against a wall, bent at a 90-degree angle..
2. Extend your arms out to the sides for support.
3. Slowly lower both legs towards the floor to your left side
4. Bring your legs back up to the starting position and repeat on your right side

COMMON MISTAKES TO AVOID

- Not alternating between legs.
- Bending your legs during the movement.
- Rushing through the exercise.

GENERAL TIPS:

- Inhale at the beginning of the movement and exhale slowly as you lower your legs towards the floor
- Avoid rushing through the exercise and focus on maintaining control throughout.

WALL SUPPORTED SQUAT + KICKBACK (60 SEC)

This is phenomenal exercise that will fire up your gluteus and quadriceps muscles.

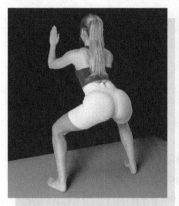
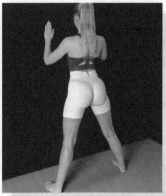
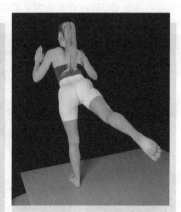
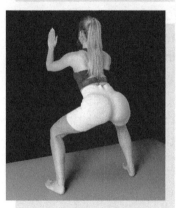
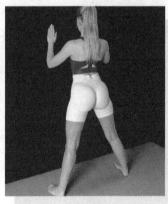
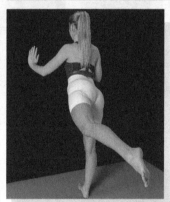

COMMON MISTAKES TO AVOID

- Allowing your elbows to flare out to the sides.
- Not lowering yourself fully to the wall
- Dropping your body instead of controlling the descent.
- Holding your breath.

GENERAL TIPS:

- Inhale deeply before starting the movement and exhale as you push yourself back up.
- Keep your core engaged and maintain a straight line from your head to your heels.

INSTRUCTIONS:

1. Stand tall facing the wall
2. Put your hands on the wall
3. Widen your stance a little bit.
4. Widen your stance a little bit
5. Squat down, go up, and kick your right leg backwards.
6. Squat down again, go up, and kick your left leg backwards

STANDING CLAMSHELLS (60 SEC)

Standing Clamshells will work onto your side glute muscles. This type of exercise will also activate your calf muscles.

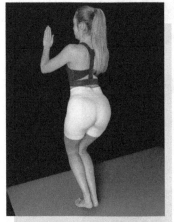
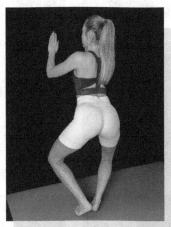
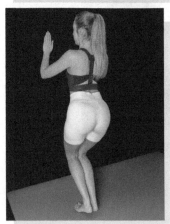

INSTRUCTIONS:

1. Stand with your back against a wall.
2. Put your hands on the wall
3. Put your hands on the wall
4. Keep your feet together and lift your heels up
5. Gently bend your knees.
6. Open your knees to the side and slowly bring them together

COMMON MISTAKES TO AVOID

- Going too fast
- Arching your spine
- Holding your breath

GENERAL TIPS:

- To make this exercise more challenging try putting resistance band above your knees
- Focus on maintaining control throughout the movement.

SINGLE LEG GLUTE BRIDGE (LEFT) (60 SEC)

Single Leg Glute Bridge will strengthen your hamstrings and glute muscles. This exercise will also improve your external hip mobility.

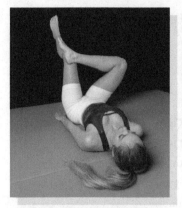 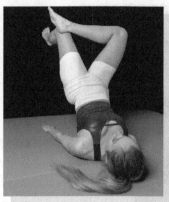

INSTRUCTIONS:

1. Lay down on the floor and engage your core.
2. Put your left leg on the wall bent at 90-degree angle.
3. Put your right ankle over your left knee.
4. From here, lift your hips up.
5. Slowly go down.

COMMON MISTAKES TO AVOID:

- Holding your breath.
- Not engaging your core.
- Excessively arching your spine.

GENERAL TIPS:

- inhale at the beginning of the movement, and slowly exhale as you start lifting your hips up.

SINGLE LEG GLUTE BRIDGE (RIGHT) (60 SEC)

Single Leg Glute Bridge will strengthen your hamstrings and glute muscles. This exercise will also improve your external hip mobility.

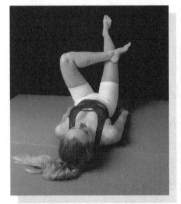
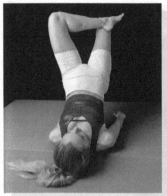
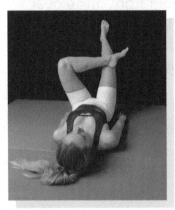

INSTRUCTIONS:

1. Lay down on the floor and engage your core.
2. Put your left right on the wall bent at 90-degree angle.
3. Put your left ankle over your right knee.
4. From here, lift your hips up.
5. Slowly go down.

COMMON MISTAKES TO AVOID:

- Holding your breath.
- Not engaging your core.
- Excessively arching your spine.

GENERAL TIPS:

- inhale at the beginning of the movement, and slowly exhale as you start lifting your hips up.

WALL SUPPORTED LATERAL SQUAT (60 SEC)

Wall Supported Lateral Squats. strengthens the quadriceps and glute muscles.

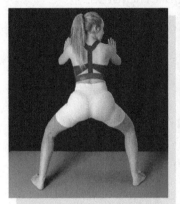
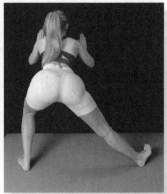
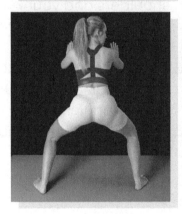
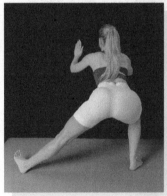

INSTRUCTIONS:

1. Stand facing a wall with your hands on it for support.
2. Keep your feet wider than hip-width apart and turn your toes out slightly.
3. Squat down and do a pulse squat on your right leg, while keeping your left leg extended to the side.
4. Alternate between legs.

COMMON MISTAKES TO AVOID

- Holding your breath.
- Rushing the movement.
- Not alternating between sides.

GENERAL TIPS:

- Inhale at the top of the movement.
- Exhale as you end the squat.

FIRE HYDRANT (RIGHT) (60 SEC)

The following exercise will help to realign hips and strengthen glutes.

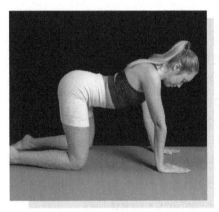 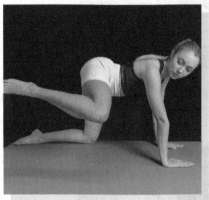

INSTRUCTIONS:

1. Begin on all fours with your hands beneath your shoulders and your knees and hips at a 90-degree angle.
2. Lift your right knee to the side, keeping it at a 90-degree angle.
3. Return your knee to the starting position and repeat.

COMMON MISTAKES TO AVOID

- Do not overextend your hip and make sure to keep your core engaged
- Do not twist your hips to raise your leg higher.
- Rushing the movement, which can compromise your form and reduce its effectiveness.

GENERAL TIPS:

- Don't worry too much about raising your leg really high. Instead, think about keeping your core engaged and in proper alignment.
- The more you practice, the better your range of motion will become

FIRE HYDRANT (LEFT) (60 SEC)

The following exercise will help to realign hips and strengthen glutes.

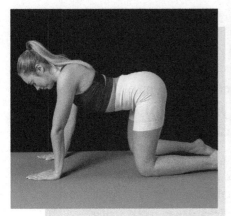
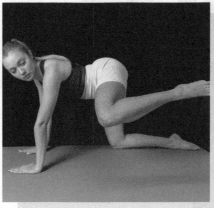

INSTRUCTIONS:

1. Begin on all fours with your hands beneath your shoulders and your knees and hips at a 90-degree angle.
2. Lift your left knee to the side, keeping it at a 90-degree angle.
3. Return your knee to the starting position and repeat..

COMMON MISTAKES TO AVOID

- Do not overextend your hip and make sure to keep your core engaged
- Do not twist your hips to raise your leg higher.
- Rushing the movement, which can compromise your form and reduce its effectiveness.

GENERAL TIPS:

- Don't worry too much about raising your leg really high. Instead, think about keeping your core engaged and in proper alignment.
- The more you practice, the better your range of motion will become.

STANDING SIDE KICK (RIGHT) (60 SEC)

standing side kick is an exercise that targets can activates your glutes muscles and help build strength in that area.

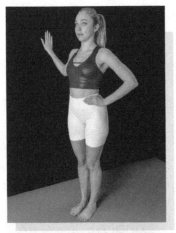
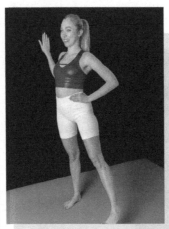
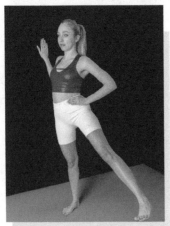

INSTRUCTIONS:

1. Stand sideways to the wall with your left hand on the wall and right hand on your hip.
2. Keep your feet together.
3. Without bending your body, kick sideways with your right leg.

COMMON MISTAKES TO AVOID

- Bending your knees.
- Allowing your body to bend while kicking sideways.
- Holding your breath.

GENERAL TIPS:

- Keep your core engaged and avoid leaning to the opposite side.
- Focus on lifting your leg with control, rather than swinging it.

STANDING SIDE KICK (LEFT) (60 SEC)

standing side kick is an exercise that targets can activates your glutes muscles and help build strength in that area.

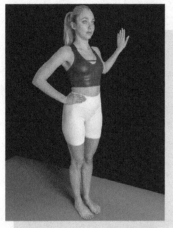
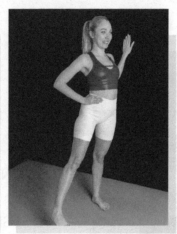
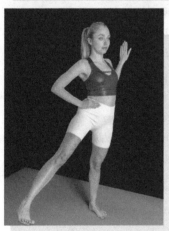

INSTRUCTIONS:

1. Stand sideways to the wall with your right hand on the wall and left hand on your hip.
2. Keep your feet together.
3. Without bending your body, kick sideways with your left leg.

COMMON MISTAKES TO AVOID

- Bending your knees.
- Allowing your body to bend while kicking sideways.
- Holding your breath.

GENERAL TIPS:

- Keep your core engaged and avoid leaning to the opposite side.
- Focus on lifting your leg with control, rather than swinging it.

STANCE CHANGING SQUAT (60 SEC)

This exercise stretches your hamstrings and calve muscles. It will mobilize your lower and upper back.

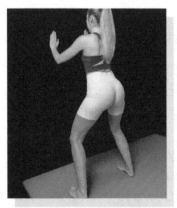
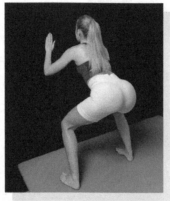
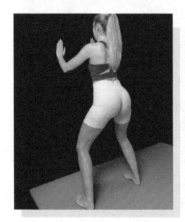
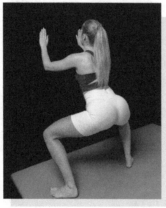

INSTRUCTIONS:

1. Stand a little bit away from the wall.
2. Put your hands on the wall
3. Take a bit wider stance
4. Squat down, and as you are coming up rotate your feet and
5. knees outwards
6. Squat down again and return to previous position.

COMMON MISTAKES TO AVOID

- Arching your back
- Holding the breath
- Rushing the movement

GENERAL TIPS:

- Inhale at the top of the movement, and exhale as you are ending the squat.

WALL SIT WITH LEG EXTENSION (60 SEC)

This is fantastic exercise that will strengthen your lower body muscles. It will also strengthen your quadriceps tendons.

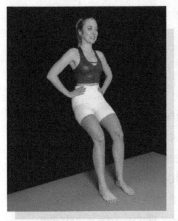
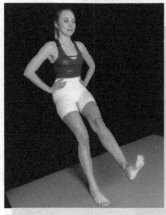
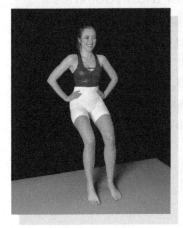
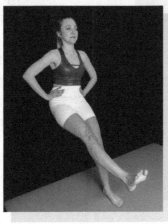

INSTRUCTIONS:

1. Put your upper back against the wall
2. Squat down until your knees are bent at a 90-degrees angle.
3. While sitting in this position, lift and extend one of your legs.
4. Alternate between the legs

COMMON MISTAKES TO AVOID

- Rushing the movement.
- Not going down to 90-degrees.
- Holding your breath.

GENERAL TIPS:

- Do not hold your breath while doing this exercise, maintain regular breathing pattern while doing this exercise
.

ELEVATED GLUTE BRIDGE + CLAM SHELL (60 SEC)

This is a fantastic exercise that targets your glutes and hamstrings.

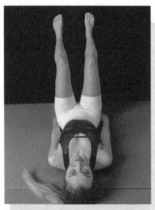
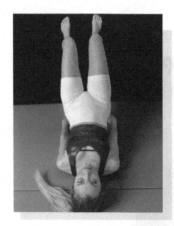
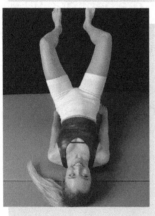

INSTRUCTIONS:

1. Lie on your back with your feet on the wall and your knees bent at a 90-degree angle.
2. Place your feet slightly higher than your knees.
3. Raise your hips up into a glute bridge position.
4. While keeping your hips lifted, open your knees to the side, then close them again.

COMMON MISTAKES TO AVOID

- Arching your back too much.
- Rushing the movement.
- Holding your breath.

GENERAL TIPS:

- Exhale as you open your knees and inhale as you close them.
- Focus on keeping your core engaged and your back flat on the ground.

DYNAMIC HIP FLEXOR STRETCH (LEFT) (60 SEC)

Dynamic hip flexor stretch is an effective exercise to dynamically strengthen your legs and it stretch your hip flexor muscles

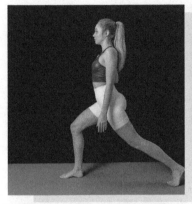 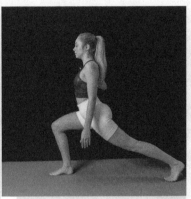

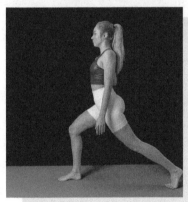

INSTRUCTIONS:

1. Stand sideways of the wall.
2. Put your right hand on the wall.
3. Keep your feet together.
4. Make a long backwards lunge with your left leg, and keep it straight the whole time.
5. Perform pulses in this lunged position.

COMMON MISTAKES TO AVOID

- Keeping your backwards leg extended
- Holding your breath
- Excessively arching your back

GENERAL TIPS:

- Do not hold your breath while doing this exercise, maintain regular breathing pattern while doing this exercise.

DYNAMIC HIP FLEXOR STRETCH (RIGHT) (60 SEC)

Dynamic hip flexor stretch is an effective exercise to dynamically strengthen your legs and it stretch your hip flexor muscles

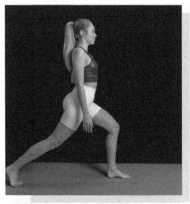
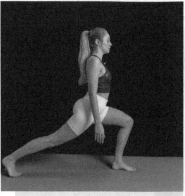
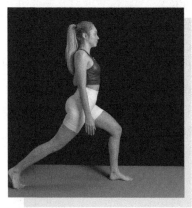

INSTRUCTIONS:

1. Stand sideways of the wall.
2. Put your left hand on the wall.
3. Keep your feet together.
4. Make a long backwards lunge with your right leg, and keep it straight the whole time.
5. Perform pulses in this lunged position.

COMMON MISTAKES TO AVOID

- Keeping your backwards leg extended
- Holding your breath
- Excessively arching your back

GENERAL TIPS:

- Do not hold your breath while doing this exercise, maintain regular breathing pattern while doing this exercise.

DYNAMIC BACKWARD LUNGE (RIGHT) (60 SEC)

This exercise is designed to work onto your quadriceps and glute muscles. It will also activate your hip flexor muscles

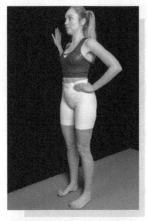 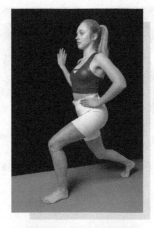 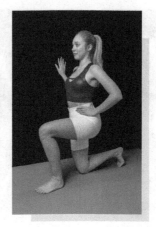

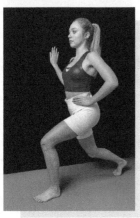 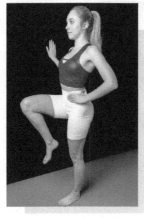

INSTRUCTIONS:

1. Stand sideways of the wall
2. Keep your feet together.
3. Put your right hand on the wall and your left one on the hip.
4. Lunge backwards with your right leg.
5. When your knee touches the floor go back and lift your right knee up.

COMMON MISTAKES TO AVOID

- Arching your spine.
- Reducing range of motion.
- Holding your breath.

GENERAL TIPS:

- Inhale before you start lunging, and slowly exhale as you start doing so.

DYNAMIC BACKWARD LUNGE (LEFT) (60 SEC)

This exercise is designed to work onto your quadriceps and glute muscles. It will also activate your hip flexor muscles

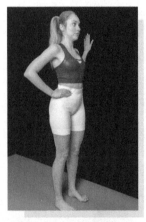 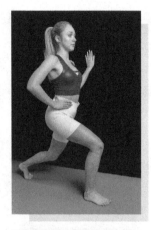 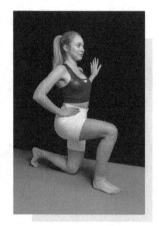

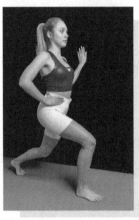 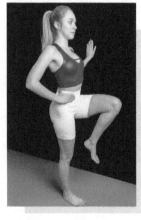

INSTRUCTIONS:

1. Stand sideways of the wall
2. Keep your feet together.
3. Put your right hand on the wall and your right one on the hip.
4. Lunge backwards with your left leg.
5. When your knee touches the floor go back and lift your left knee up.

COMMON MISTAKES TO AVOID

- Arching your spine.
- Reducing range of motion.
- Holding your breath.

GENERAL TIPS:

- Inhale before you start lunging, and slowly exhale as you start doing so.

ELEVATED GLUTE BRIDGE (60 SEC)

Elevated Glute Bridge is excellent exercise that will work on your hamstring and glute muscles

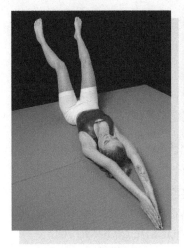 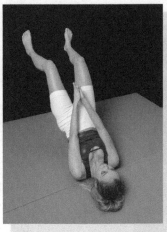

INSTRUCTIONS:

1. Lay on your back.
2. Put your feet on the wall with a bit wider stance.
3. Put your hands together above your head.
4. Lift your hips up, and bring your hands towards your lower abdomen.
5. Slowly go back to starting position.

COMMON MISTAKES TO AVOID

- Not keeping your core engaged.
- Holding your breath.
- Excessively arching your lower back.

GENERAL TIPS:

- Make sure to keep your core flexed. Doing this will eliminate the stress on your lower back.

WALL SHOULDER TAPS (60 SEC)

Wall Shoulder Taps are a great exercise that will improve your shoulder stability with minimal effort on the whole body.

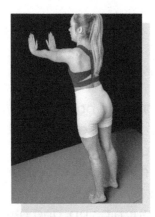
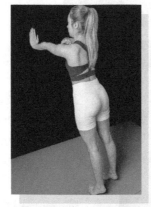
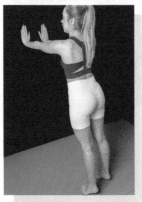
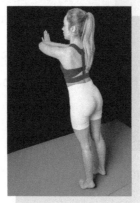

INSTRUCTIONS:

1. Stand tall a step or two away from the wall, while facing it.
2. Put your hands on the wall at your shoulder level.
3. Keep your feet together.
4. Touch your right shoulder with your left hand.
5. Alternate between sides.

COMMON MISTAKES TO AVOID

- Not alternating between sides
- Holding your breath
- Arching your spine
- Not keeping your core engaged

GENERAL TIPS:

- Maintain a regular breathing pattern while performing this exercise. Ensure that your core is engaged throughout the movement.

WALL SIT CALF RAISES (60 SEC)

Wall Sit Calf Raises will strengthen your calve muscles and quadriceps muscles as well. This exercise will also strengthen your ankles and quadriceps tendons.

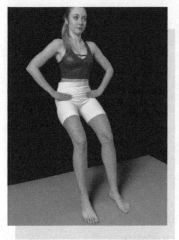
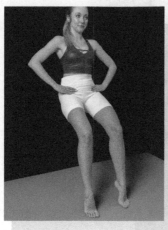

INSTRUCTIONS:

1. Put your upper back against the wall.
2. Squat down until your knees are bent at a 90-degrees angle.
3. While sitting in this position, lift your heels up by pressing your toes to the floor.
4. Slowly bring them down.

COMMON MISTAKES TO AVOID

- Holding your breath
- Rushing the movement
- Letting your upper back off the wall

GENERAL TIPS:

- Do not hold your breath while doing this exercise, maintain regular breathing pattern.

CHEST WALL PUSH UPS (60 SEC)

Chest Wall Push Up is great exercise that will blow up your chest and triceps muscles. It is also good way to condition your tendons for heavier variations of push ups.

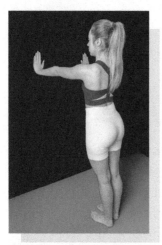 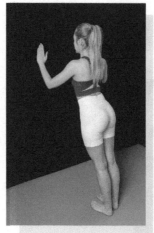

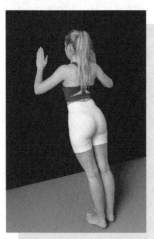

INSTRUCTIONS:

1. Stand tall with your feet a bit narrower.
2. Put your hands onto the wall at your chest level
3. Keep your elbows at 45-degrees angle.
4. From there, lower yourself until your chest touches the wall.
5. Push yourself up.

COMMON MISTAKES TO AVOID

- Not keeping your elbows at 45-degrees angle.
- Partial range of motion.
- Holding the breath.

GENERAL TIPS:

- Inhale at the beginning of the movement, and slowly exhale as you push yourself up.
- Always keep your elbows at 45-degrees angle.

ABDOMINAL TWIST (60 SEC)

This exercise stretches your spinal erector muscles and work your side abdominal muscles.

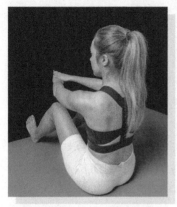
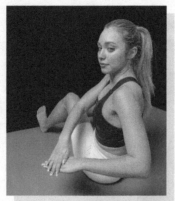
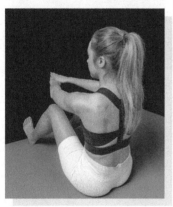
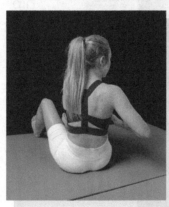

INSTRUCTIONS:

1. Sit down and put your feet on the wall.
2. Keep your knees slightly bent and lean a bit backwards.
3. Put your hands together in front of you.
4. From here, twist your body to one side, and touch down the floor with your hands.
5. Alternate between sides.

COMMON MISTAKES TO AVOID

- Holding your breath
- Not touching the floor with your hands
- Rotating too slowly.

GENERAL TIPS:

- Inhale at the beginning of the movement, and slowly exhale as the movement continues.
- Maintain a steady breathing pattern throughout the exercise.

STANDING SIDE KICK (RIGHT) (60 SEC)

standing side kick is an exercise that targets can activates your glutes muscles and help build strength in that area.

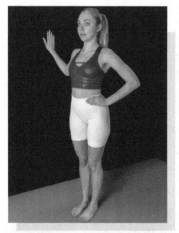
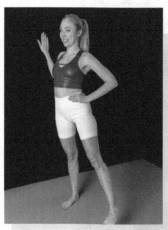
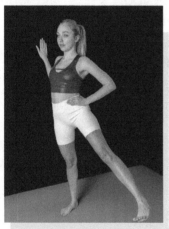

INSTRUCTIONS:

1. Stand sideways to the wall with your left hand on the wall and right hand on your hip.
2. Keep your feet together.
3. Without bending your body, kick sideways with your right leg.

COMMON MISTAKES TO AVOID

- Bending your knees.
- Allowing your body to bend while kicking sideways.
- Holding your breath.

GENERAL TIPS:

- Keep your core engaged and avoid leaning to the opposite side.
- Focus on lifting your leg with control, rather than swinging it.

STANDING SIDE KICK (LEFT) (60 SEC)

standing side kick is an exercise that targets can activates your glutes muscles and help build strength in that area.

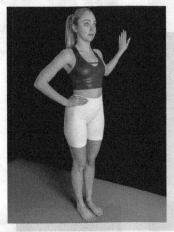
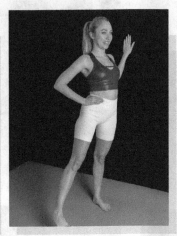
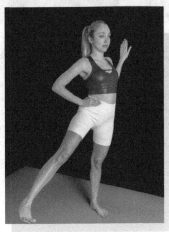

INSTRUCTIONS:

1. Stand sideways to the wall with your right hand on the wall and left hand on your hip.
2. Keep your feet together.
3. Without bending your body, kick sideways with your left leg.

COMMON MISTAKES TO AVOID

- Bending your knees.
- Allowing your body to bend while kicking sideways.
- Holding your breath.

GENERAL TIPS:

- Keep your core engaged and avoid leaning to the opposite side.
- Focus on lifting your leg with control, rather than swinging it.

WALL PUSH UP PLANK (60 SEC)

Wall Push up Plank is interesting exercise that will warm up and strengthen your triceps and shoulder muscles.

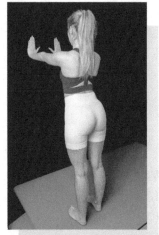 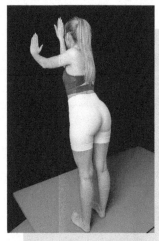 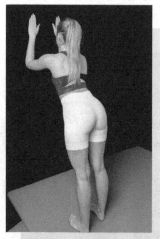 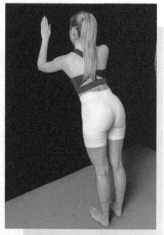

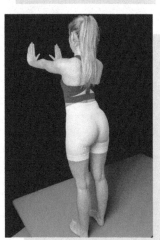 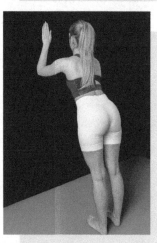 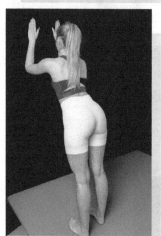 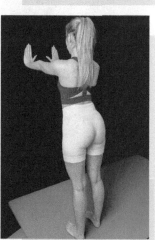

COMMON MISTAKES TO AVOID

- Excessively arching your spine
- Rushing the movement
- Holding your breath

GENERAL TIPS:

- Maintain a regular breathing pattern.
- Focus on performing the exercise with control and without rushing through the motion.

INSTRUCTIONS:

1. Stand tall step or two away from the wall, while facing it.
2. Put your hands on the wall and keep your feet together.
3. While keeping your arms extended, bend your right elbow, and then bend your left elbow
4. Reverse the movement into starting position.

CALF RAISED SQUAT (60 SEC)

Calf Raised Squat is an effective exercise that will activate your whole lower body muscles and increase your stability.

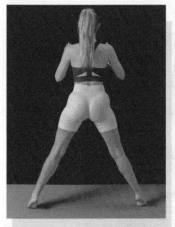
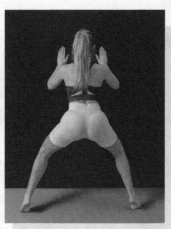
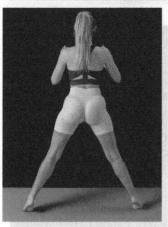

INSTRUCTIONS:

1. Stand on your toes facing the wall
2. Put both hands on the wall
3. Make sure your stance is wider and your knees are pointing outwards
4. Slowly squat down until your knees are bent at 90 degrees
5. Keep your back straight during the entire exercise.

COMMON MISTAKES TO AVOID

- Arching your spine.
- Holding your breath.
- Not going down to 90-degrees.

GENERAL TIPS:

- Inhale at the top of the movement, engage your stomach muscles, squat down and exhale as you go up.

WALL SUPPORTED BICYCLE CRUNCH (60 SEC)

Wall Supported Bicycle Crunch is fantastic exercise that will fire up you whole abdominal muscles.

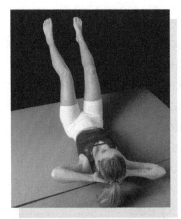 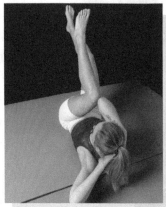 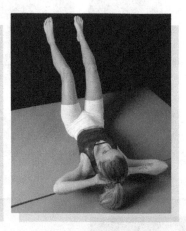

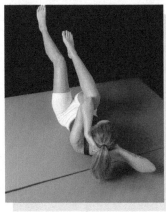

INSTRUCTIONS:

1. Lay on the floor with your feet on the wall.
2. Keep your legs extended on the wall.
3. Put your hands behind your head.
4. Crunch up, and with your left elbow touch your right knee, while tucking it. towards your chest
5. Do both sides.

COMMON MISTAKES TO AVOID

- Not alternating between sides
- Holding your breath
- Using momentum

GENERAL TIPS:

- Inhale at the beginning of the movement, and slowly exhale as you start crunching up.

SINGLE LEG GLUTE BRIDGE (LEFT) (60 SEC)

Single Leg Glute Bridge will strengthen your hamstrings and glute muscles. This exercise will also improve your external hip mobility.

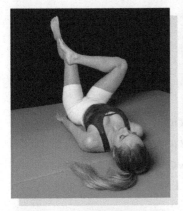
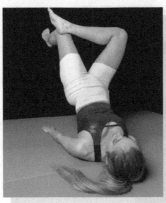
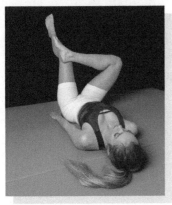

INSTRUCTIONS:

1. Lay down on the floor and engage your core.
2. Put your left leg on the wall bent at 90-degree angle.
3. Put your right ankle over your left knee.
4. From here, lift your hips up.
5. Slowly go down.

COMMON MISTAKES TO AVOID:

- Holding your breath.
- Not engaging your core.
- Excessively arching your spine.

GENERAL TIPS:

- inhale at the beginning of the movement, and slowly exhale as you start lifting your hips up.

SINGLE LEG GLUTE BRIDGE (RIGHT) (60 SEC)

Single Leg Glute Bridge will strengthen your hamstrings and glute muscles. This exercise will also improve your external hip mobility.

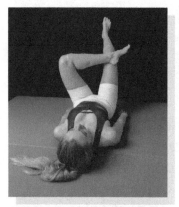 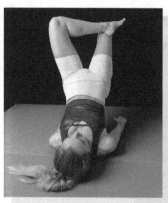

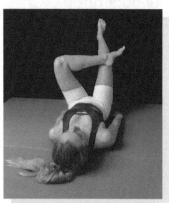

INSTRUCTIONS:

1. Lay down on the floor and engage your core.
2. Put your left right on the wall bent at 90-degree angle.
3. Put your left ankle over your right knee.
4. From here, lift your hips up.
5. Slowly go down.

COMMON MISTAKES TO AVOID:

- Holding your breath.
- Not engaging your core.
- Excessively arching your spine.

GENERAL TIPS:

- inhale at the beginning of the movement, and slowly exhale as you start lifting your hips up.

OTHER TIPS TO KEEP YOU HEALTHY!

NUTRITION

Nutrition is one of the best ways of preserving your health and overall wellbeing. It is the process by which the body obtains and utilizes essential nutrients from food to support growth, maintenance, and repair of body tissues. A balanced diet that provides all the necessary nutrients is crucial for maintaining optimal health and preventing chronic diseases. What is also important is to consider the effects of bad nutrition :

EFFECTS	CONSEQUENCES
POOR IMMUNE SYSTEM	Impaired ability to fight infection
REDUCED MUSCLE STRENGTH AND FATIGUE	Reduced capacity to work, shop, cook, and take care of oneself due to inactivity. The poor muscular function can lead to falls, and poor respiratory muscle function can lead to low cough pressure, which can delay expectoration and recovery from a chest infection.
IMPAIRED WOUND HEALING	Infections and un-united fractures are more common as a result of increased wound-related complications.
IMPAIRED PSYCHO-SOCIAL FUNCTION	Malnutrition causes apathy, sadness, introversion, self-neglect, hypochondriasis, loss of libido, and worsening in social relations.

Nutrition preserves your health by providing all the nutrients your body needs in order to function properly. The body needs a variety of different nutrients to maintain the health and strength of your bones, muscles, organs, connective tissues and so much more. This is why a balanced diet is so important.

Every nutrient performs a different role within the body, and each nutrient is codependent. This means that if you don't obtain enough of one nutrient, the body will struggle to absorb another. This can create a ripple effect leading to numerous nutritional deficiencies. Then, these deficiencies can cause symptoms like weak bones, tiredness, mood swings, hormonal imbalances, and more.

So, how do you ensure that you eat healthily? The Eatwell Guide sets out food categories and recommendations for all. By consuming a mixture of all food groups, you will consume a variety of nutrients required to keep you healthy.

FRUIT AND VEGETABLES

39% of our total food intake should come from fruit and vegetables. This can be translated into consuming 5 portions of fruit and vegetables per day.

A portion is:
- Approximately 80g of fruit
- 1 whole medium-sized piece of fruit eg. Apple/banana
- 2 small-sized pieces of fruit eg. Satsuma/plum
- 1 large slice of pineapple/melon
- 3 tablespoons of vegetables
- 1desert sized bowl of salad
- 30g dried fruit
- 150mls unsweetened fruit juice
- 150mls smoothie

Fresh, frozen, tinned, and dried fruit all count towards our 5 a day. If you are underweight or you've experienced significant weight loss in a short period of time then tinned fruit in syrup would be more sensible. We should aim to eat a variety of different coloured fruits and vegetables as they contain different antioxidants. The main nutrients provided in fruit include dietary fibre, vitamin C, potassium, folate and vitamin A.

STARCHY CARBOHYDRATES

37% of your total food intake should come from starchy carbohydrates.

Good examples of carbohydrates include:
- Breakfast cereals
- Couscous
- Semolina
- Tapioca
- Bulgar wheat.

Starchy foods should ideally be included at every mealtime. Wholegrain and wholemeal versions should be chosen where possible to help meet your fibre requirements of 30 grams per day. This is especially important for older people due to higher occurrences of constipation. Starchy carbohydrates provide dietary fibre, B vitamins, carbs, and calcium.

PROTEIN

On average, a middle aged person requires approximately 0.75g of protein per kilogram of body weight a day/ However, many adults need 1g of protein per kg of bodyweight. The intake can also be different depending on your nutritional status and weight. Approximately 12-15% of our total food intake should come from this section. Beans, peas, tofu, lentils, and other vegetables are a good source of alternatives to meat as they are low in fat and high in protein, vitamins, and minerals.

It is recommended that adults eat two portions of fish per week, one of which should be oily such as salmon or herring. These oily fish are a valuable source of omega 3 fatty acids which can have a positive effect on memory, heart health and inflammation, and mood.

These foods are a good source of iron, which is essential for making red blood cells that carry oxygen around the body. A lack of iron can lead to iron deficiency anemia. This is common in older individuals as its prevalence increases with age. This can also occur as a result of chronic gastrointestinal blood loss caused by some medications and gut conditions. This type of anemia should be treated with iron supplements. On average an older adult requires 8.7mg per day. Those with a diagnosed deficiency require more and should be managed by a medical professional. This food group provides nutrients like iron, protein, b vitamins, and omega 3 fats.

FATS, SALT, AND SUGAR

Foods high in sugar, salt, and fat such as biscuits, cakes, and soft drinks sit outside the Eatwell Guide. While these foods can be enjoyed in moderation as part of a balanced diet, if eaten regularly they can increase the risk of health conditions such as high blood pressure, obesity, and type 2 diabetes. It is also important to stay hydrated, try to drink 6-8 glasses of fluids daily.

DAIRY AND ALTERNATIVES

8% of your total food intake should come from this section. Milk, cheese, and yogurt are excellent sources of calcium and protein and we should aim to eat 3 portions every day.

Great sources include 200ml of milk, a pot of yoghurt or a matchbox size of cheese as well as calcium-enriched alternative milk like almond, rice and soya. This food group provides nutrients like calcium, protein, vitamin A.

OILS AND SPREADS

Oils and spreads can be high in saturated fats so it's important to minimise these and choose healthier choices. These include plant sources like rapeseed, sunflower, or olive oil. Unsaturated fats are more cardio-protective (heart-healthy) than saturated versions like butter and lard.

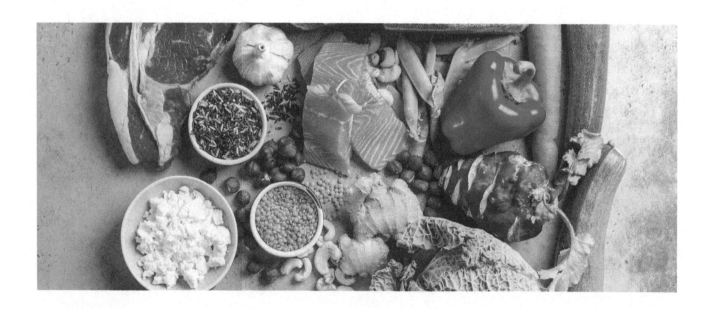

CALORIE AND MACRO REQUIREMENTS

Below is a table that summarises calorie and macronutrients requirements for average persons in different age categories.

AGE	30-59		60-75	
NUTRIENT	MALE	FEMALE	MALE	FEMALE
CALORIES	2,590	1,912	2,210	1,930
PROTEIN (G/DAY)*	0.7xKg	0.7xKg	1.1xKg	1.1xKg
TOTAL FAT (G/DAY)	~80	~59	~68	~59
CARBOHYDRATES** (G/DAY)	~324	~239	~277	~242
FIBRE (G/DAY)	~30	~30	~30	~30

These are recommended intakes for average persons and can vary based on a persons body composition and health.

* These are recommended intakes for average persons and it is calculated based per each Kg of you the total body weight (example weight: 75 kg male proteins: 0.7 x 75KG = 52.5 gr of proteins)

** the g/day recommended sugars intakes is averagely the 10% of the carbohydrates

VITAMINS AND MINERALS IMPORTANT FOR SENIORS

Everything we eat should be packed with nutrients in order to achieve the recommended intake.

There are certain nutrients that are more important than others, especially when we get older.

CALCIUM

Calcium is vital for maintaining healthy bones and teeth. This nutrient can be obtained from dairy products and alternatives.

VITAMIN D

Vitamin D aids in the absorption of calcium, the maintenance of bone density, and the prevention of osteoporosis. Vitamin D has also been shown to protect against cancer, type 1 diabetes, rheumatoid arthritis, multiple sclerosis, and autoimmune illnesses in some studies. Vitamin D insufficiency has also been related to an increased risk of falling in the elderly.

VITAMIN B12

Vitamin B12 is a nutrient that aids in the health of the body's nerve and blood cells, as well as the production of DNA, which is the genetic material found in all cells. Vitamin B12 also protects against megaloblastic anaemia, which causes fatigue and weakness.

OMEGA-3 FATS

These unsaturated fats, which are mostly found in fish, may help with rheumatoid arthritis symptoms and decrease the advancement of age-related macular degeneration (AMD), a disease that causes visual loss in the elderly.

MAGNESIUM

Magnesium is involved in more than 300 different physiological activities. Getting enough can help you maintain a healthy immune system, a healthy heart, and strong bones. Older adults who use certain medications, such as diuretics, may have trouble absorbing magnesium, so a supplement may be beneficial.

FIBER

Fibre is an important nutrient that supports a healthy gut and lowers blood pressure and blood sugar. As you age, you might find that constipation can be a regular problem, obtaining enough fibre may help with this issue.

POTASSIUM

Potassium is an important mineral that helps to maintain strong bones and teeth. This mineral is necessary for cell function and has been found to help lower blood pressure and minimise the chance of kidney stones.

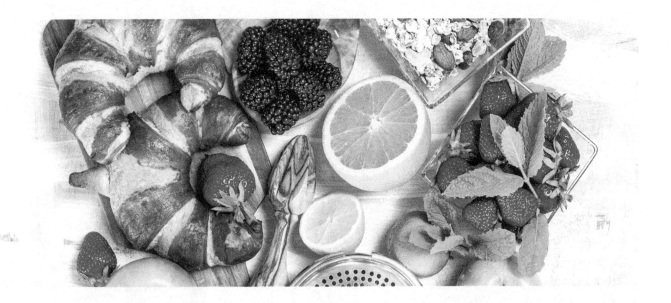

VITAMIN AND MINERALS

Below is a table that summarises vitamin and mineral requirements for average persons in different age categories.

AGE	30-59		60-75	
NUTRIENT	MALE	FEMALE	MALE	FEMALE
Vitamin A (µg/day)	700	600	700	600
Thiamin (mg/day)	1	0.9	0.9	0.7
Riboflavin (mg/day)	1.3	1.1	1.3	1.1
Niacin equivalent (mg/day)	14	14	15.1	12.1
Vitamin B6 (mg/day)	1.1	1.1	1.4	1.3
Vitamin B12 (µg/day)	2	2	1.5	1.5
Folate (µG/day)	320	320	200	200
Vitamin C (mg/day)	75	60	40	40
Vitamin D (µg/day)	10	10	10	10

µg = micrograms

MENTAL HEALTH

Maintaining good mental health in is essential for wellbeing and quality of life. Thankfully, there are a number of simple tips and strategies that can be used to help maintain mental health. In this section of the chapter, we'll look at 10 easy tips for better mental health. From activities to help reduce stress, to tips for staying connected to loved ones, these tips can make a big difference in the lives of seniors.

WHAT IS MENTAL HEALTH ALL ABOUT?

Mental health is more than simply being free from mental illness. It is about feeling good about yourself, having positive relationships with those around you, and coping with life's challenges in a healthy way. Mental health is an essential part of overall wellbeing, as it enables us to maintain resilience and cope with life's ups and downs. Mental health involves many aspects, including our emotions, thoughts, behaviors, and social connections.

For middle aged people but generally for everyone, it is important to stay on top of their mental health and wellbeing. Regular physical activity, social interaction, and engaging in meaningful activities can all help seniors stay mentally healthy.

BENEFITS OF TAKING CARE OF MENTAL HEALTH

Mental health is an important part of overall wellbeing, and it can become more important as we age. Taking the time to maintain good mental health can provide a number of benefits that can improve quality of life for seniors.

Some of the benefits of taking care of mental health include:
- Increased self-esteem and sense of purpose: Keeping your mind active can give you a greater sense of self-worth and help keep boredom at bay.
- Improved social connections: Connecting with others can help reduce feelings of loneliness and isolation, and make life more enjoyable.

- Reduced stress: Lowering stress levels can reduce anxiety and depression symptoms, as well as improve physical health.
- Enhanced memory and cognitive functioning: Keeping your mind active can help protect against age-related cognitive decline and dementia.
- Improved mood and energy levels: Maintaining good mental health can provide a better outlook on life, as well as increase motivation to complete tasks.

Taking the time to prioritize your mental health can go a long way in providing positive benefits to your overall wellbeing. These benefits may include improved quality of life and better overall physical health.

TIPS FOR BETTER MENTAL HEALTH

GO FOR REGULAR WALKS AND FRESH AIR

Regular exercise is important for physical and mental health. Going for walks can be a great way for everyone to get the exercise they need and get some fresh air at the same time. Fresh air can do wonders for your mental health and going on a walk can help you clear your head, reduce stress, and improve your mood. If possible, try to walk in a park or other outdoor area with plenty of greenery and nature. This can help you relax and enjoy the scenery while you're walking. For those who have difficulty getting out and walking, joining a walking group may be an option. Walking groups provide companionship, accountability, and encouragement to help seniors get the exercise they need.

GET ENOUGH SLEEP

Sleep is an important part of keeping good mental health, and seniors are no exception. A lack of quality sleep can lead to depression, anxiety, cognitive decline, and many other issues.

The National Institute on Aging recommends that seniors aim for seven to nine hours of sleep every night. However, if you find yourself struggling to stay asleep or get enough restorative sleep, you may need to adjust your sleeping habits.

For starters, try to go to bed and wake up at the same time every day. Create a relaxing nighttime routine by dimming the lights and avoiding screens for at least an hour before bed. It's also important to keep your bedroom cool and comfortable—around 65°F is ideal—and to limit caffeine and alcohol consumption in the evening.

If you're still having trouble sleeping, talk to your doctor about possible treatments, such as cognitive-behavioral therapy (CBT), natural supplements or medications that may help you get better rest. With the right steps, you can make sure you're getting enough sleep each night and taking care of your mental health.

TAKE BREAKS DURING THE DAY

Taking breaks during the day can help stay focused and keep their mental health in check. Even if it's just taking a few minutes to sit and relax, stepping away from your work or day-to-day activities can be beneficial. Taking a short walk outside, listening to some calming music, or reading a book are all good ways to take a break during the day.

If possible, try to create a set schedule where you can plan regular breaks throughout the day. During these breaks, make sure to step away from screens and electronics and engage in some sort of activity that will help to reduce stress. This could be something as simple as stretching, meditating, deep breathing exercises, or yoga.

If you have a hard time remembering to take breaks throughout the day, try setting a reminder on your phone or computer. You may also want to ask family members or friends to remind you when it's time for a break. Taking time for yourself can help you remain focused and energized for whatever tasks come next.

CONNECT WITH OTHERS

Staying socially connected is important for all of us, especially older people. Social interaction helps to stimulate the mind and maintain a healthy emotional state. Make time to reach out and connect with friends, family members, and even strangers. This could be as simple as taking a walk around the block and saying hello to your neighbors or joining an online forum. If you are feeling more adventurous, you could join a local club or organization, volunteer at a charity event, or simply make plans to have lunch with an old friend.

No matter how you choose to stay connected, remember that social interaction can be very beneficial for mental health. It helps to increase feelings of belonging, provide support during difficult times, and can even help reduce stress and anxiety. It is essential that we make time in our lives for meaningful relationships and activities that bring us joy and purpose.

DO SOMETHING YOU ENJOY EVERY DAY

It's important for to make time for activities to get your mind and body activated. Doing something you enjoy every day can be a great way to boost your mental health and overall wellbeing. Whether it's reading a book, doing a craft, going for a bike ride, or having coffee with a friend, it's important to make time for things that bring you happiness.

Having an activity that you look forward to every day can be an incredible source of joy and comfort, especially during times when it can be difficult to stay positive. It's also a great way to stay active and social, which are key to maintaining good mental health in seniors.

The important thing is to find something that brings you joy. It doesn't have to be anything big or complicated – it could be as simple as spending 10 minutes playing with a pet, or watching your favorite show. The goal is to do something that makes you feel happy and relaxed, so you can focus on the positive aspects of life.

VOLUNTEER

Volunteering is a great way for seniors to give back and help their community. It can also be beneficial to their mental health by providing a sense of purpose, making them feel needed, and increasing their social interaction.

For those who are physically able, they can participate in tasks such as gardening, visiting the elderly, or helping with home repairs. For those who are not as mobile, there are still plenty of volunteer opportunities, such as tutoring, fundraising, and working in the office. Whatever their passion may be, there is likely a volunteer opportunity that will fit it.

Another great way for older people to volunteer is through virtual volunteering. This form of volunteering allows them to stay connected with others while doing something worthwhile from the comfort of their own home. They can participate in activities such as transcribing audio files, proofreading documents, or participating in online surveys.

Volunteering has been proven to have positive impacts on mental health and overall wellbeing. It's a great way to give back while staying active and engaged with the community. With so many options available, there is something for everyone to do.

LEARN SOMETHING NEW

Learning something new is a great way to stay mentally active and engaged. Taking classes, going to lectures, joining a book club, or reading more can be great ways to explore the world and keep your mind sharp. There are many online courses and educational programs available, as well as in-person learning opportunities. Learning something new can also help seniors stay up to date with the latest technology and trends. Take the time to find something that interests you and commit to learning more about it!

BE MINDFUL OF YOUR THOUGHTS

It's important for everybody to be mindful of their thoughts. The mind can play tricks on us, often leading us to overthink and worry excessively about situations that are outside of our control. When we allow ourselves to be consumed by negative thinking, it can quickly spiral out of control.

Instead, take the time to recognize your thoughts and choose how to respond to them. Remind yourself that thoughts are not facts, and that you have the power to choose which ones to hold on to. Take a few moments to pause and be present in the moment without judgment or expectation. Acknowledge any negative thoughts, but also make an effort to reframe them in a more positive light.

When facing mental health struggles, it can be helpful to seek out professional help from a therapist or doctor. Remember that these issues should not be taken lightly, and there is no shame in asking for support. Mental health issues can affect anyone at any age, so don't hesitate to reach out for help if needed.

SEEK PROFESSIONAL HELP IF NEEDED

Mental health issues can be difficult to manage on your own, so it's important to seek professional help if needed. Consulting a mental health specialist such as a psychologist can be beneficial for everybody who are having difficulty coping with emotional challenges. There are also many services available that provide support, counseling, and other forms of assistance. It is important to remember that seeking professional help is not a sign of weakness, but rather a sign of strength and courage. Taking the steps necessary to get the help you need is an important step in maintaining good mental health.

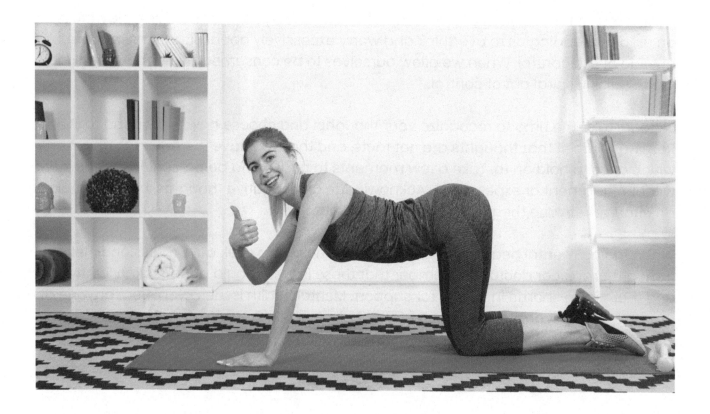

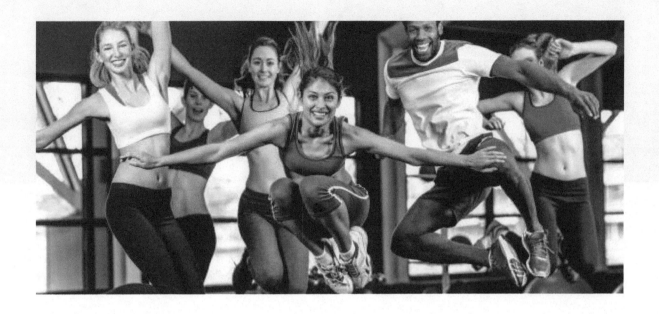

T H A N K   Y O U !

At the end of the day, wall pilates for has proven itself to be an invaluable form of exercise that can truly improve the overall health.
wall pilates can truly be considered a "gift of health" enabling everybody to reach their physical, mental, and emotional goals while having fun and feeling healthier.
Thank you so much for choosing our guide to help you achieve optimum health. We hope you've enjoyed the content!

If so, I have a small request for you.

If you've found value in your reading experience today, I humbly ask that you take a brief moment right now to leave an honest review of this book. It won't cost you anything but 30 seconds of your time—just a few seconds to share your thoughts with others.

If you're reading on Kindle or an e-reader, simply scroll to the last page of the book and swipe up—the review should prompt from there.

If you're on a Paperback or any other physical format of this book, you can find the book page on Amazon (or wherever you bought this) and leave your review right there.

Rita Davis

Made in the USA
Coppell, TX
09 August 2023

20138552R00057